The Digest Diet

Breakthrough Science!
The Best Foods for Fast, Lasting Weight Loss

BY LIZ VACCARIELLO

Editor-in-Chief of *Reader's Digest*, coauthor of the
#1 New York Times bestseller ***Flat Belly Diet!***

with Heather Jackson

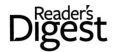

The Reader's Digest Association, Inc.
New York, NY/Montreal

PROJECT STAFF
EXECUTIVE EDITOR
Courtenay Smith
CREATIVE DIRECTOR
Robert Newman
PHOTO DIRECTOR
Bill Black
SENIOR ART DIRECTOR
George McKeon
DESIGN CONSULTANTS
Jennifer Tokarski, Rich Kershner
MANAGING EDITOR
Lorraine Burton
SENIOR EDITOR
Andrea Au Levitt
EDITORIAL ASSISTANT
Elizabeth Kelly
RECIPE DEVELOPERS
Kate Slate, Sandra Gluck,
Ruth Cousineau
FITNESS TRAINER
Matt Schwartz
COPY EDITOR
Lisa Andruscavage
INDEXER
Nan Badgett

CREDITS
TEST TEAM PORTRAITS
Erin Patrice O'Brien
PHOTOGRAPHY (Chapter 4)
Lisa Shin
PHOTOGRAPHY (Chapter 6)
Francesco Tonelli
FITNESS ILLUSTRATIONS
Josh McKibble
VIDEO (readersdigest.com/digestdiet)
Nicolas Montalvo
CLOTHING
15love Apparel, Asic, Eileen Fisher,
Lacoste, New Balance, Reebok, Ruby
Moriarty, Saucony, Worth

READER'S DIGEST ASSOCIATION, INC.
PRESIDENT AND CEO
Robert E. Guth
PRESIDENT, NORTH AMERICA
Dan Lagani
PRESIDENT AND PUBLISHER, BOOKS
Harold Clarke
ASSOCIATE PUBLISHER, BOOKS
Rosanne McManus
CHIEF CONTENT OFFICER, NORTH AMERICA
Liz Vaccariello

A READER'S DIGEST BOOK

Copyright © 2012 The Reader's Digest Association
All rights reserved. Unauthorized reproduction, in any manner, is prohibited. Reader's Digest is a registered trademark of The Reader's Digest Association, Inc.

Library of Congress
Cataloging-in-Publication Data
Vaccariello, Liz.
  The digest diet : the fast, effective, 21-day fat release plan / Liz Vaccariello and Heather Jackson.
    p. cm.
  ISBN 978-1-60652-543-2 (trade) -- ISBN 978-1-60652-544-9 (adobe) -- ISBN 978-1-60652-545-6 (e pub) -- ISBN 978-1-60652-543-2 (direct mail)
  1. Reducing diets. 2. Reducing diets--Recipes. 3. Reducing diets--Menus. 4. Reducing exercises. I. Jackson, Heather. II. Title.
  RM222.2.V254 2012
  613.2'5--dc23

                         2011053111

We are committed to both the quality of our products and the service we provide to our customers. We value your comments, so please feel free to contact us.

The Reader's Digest Association, Inc.
Adult Trade Publishing
44 South Broadway
White Plains, NY 10601

For more Reader's Digest products and information, visit our website:
rd.com (in the United States)
readersdigest.ca (in Canada)

Printed in the United States of America
1 3 5 7 9 10 8 6 4 2

This publication is designed to provide useful information to the reader on the subjects of weight loss, healthy eating, and exercise. It should not be substituted for the advice of a physician or used to alter any medical therapy or programs prescribed to you by your doctor. Be sure to consult your doctor before proceeding with any weight-loss or exercise regimen. The use of specific products in this book does not constitute an endorsement by the author or the publisher.

The Digest Diet

Go online for **EXCLUSIVE** success tools and tricks… **and it's all FREE!**

- **Guaranteed motivation** with community and support

- **Inspiring videos** full of savvy tips and insider advice from other Digest Diet participants

- **The latest news and studies** on fat releasing foods, moves, and attitudes, plus updates from the experts

- **Easy-to-use shopping lists** for each phase of the plan, customizable for your personal tastes

- **Even more delicious recipes** starring your favorite fat releasers to keep you feeling full and fabulous

- **Food and fitness journals** to help you reach your goal

- **The best jokes** and funny stuff to get you to "laugh it off" when you need it

readersdigest.com/digestdiet

facebook.com/digestdiet

Coming Soon: The Digest Diet Cookbook

Contents

Acknowledgments

Thank you doesn't begin to cover my gratitude for the vision, stamina, and creativity of Heather Jackson and Courtenay Smith, whose partnership and dedication (and early mornings and late nights) made excellence possible. (A wink and hug to Ashley Sandberg for the introduction that brought the dream team together.) I am also indebted to creative director Robert Newman for the simple beauty of the final product.

To the hardworking editors and designers who played roles large and small in supporting our test panel and researching portions of the book—not to mention keeping us on track to meet our deadlines! In particular: Elizabeth Kelly, Lorraine Burton, George McKeon, Andrea Au Levitt, Beth Dreher, Lauren Gniazdowski, Ann DiCesare, Lisa Andruscavage, Rich Kershner, and Jen Tokarski. Also, a fist bump to certified trainer Matt Schwartz, who designed the "quick burst" fat releasing workout and triple-checked it for accuracy, efficiency, and efficacy, and to registered nurse Wendy Horn, who measured and remeasured our test team members.

To a fantastic team of digital editors who brought the Digest Diet to life online and in social media: Diane Dragan, Jamele Polk, Lauren Gelman, Peri Blumberg.

For the wonderful photographs throughout this book: our photo director Bill Black and his team (I'm talking to you, Emilie Harjes and Rachel Hatch!). Also, to Erin Patrice O'Brien (for making our test panelists look and feel like rock stars), Lisa Shin (who made the newly discovered fat releasing foods look truly heroic), and Francesco Tonelli (the chef-photographer who made every recipe look its delicious best), and their hardworking teams of assistants and stylists.

For delicious recipes that had our test panel raving: Kate Slate, Sandra Gluck, and Ruth Cousineau.

To an incredible marketing and public relations team: Jacqueline Lachman, Gary Davis, Brian Carnahan, Tim Farrow, Wayne Nobes, Kathi Ramsdell, Debbie Duren, Joe Rinaldi, Caitlin O'Hare.

To Jill Armus, who was in the room at moment one. To Reader's Digest North America president Dan Lagani for his belief, support, and leadership. To Harold Clarke for thinking big from the get-go. To Marilynn Jacobs for shepherding it along its way.

My loudest shout-out I save for my executive assistant Adrienne Farr, who leapt up to be one of the first to try the Digest Diet—and went on to lose more than 50 pounds and counting (all while keeping me organized and sane as her day job)! I always knew you were a superstar, and now so does the whole world!

Finally, to Steve, Olivia, Sophia. For this. For everything.

Introduction

You'd be hard-pressed to find someone who walks around feeling more grateful than I do. Every day, I get to be a mom, a wife, a friend. I'm a sister and a daughter. An employee, a manager, a colleague. A runner and a reader. A writer, editor, and an occasional television personality. Just like you, I'm passionate about each of my roles and put my heart into all that I do.

A few years ago, when I was the editor-in-chief of *Prevention* magazine, I'd just come home from the road promoting my first book, *Flat Belly Diet!* At the time, my twin girls were about to turn four. They'd overheard me talk about my weight-loss plan quite a bit.

Now, I've always believed that food is a blessing. Not only is it our bodies' key supplier of health-promoting nutrients and energy, but it's the cornerstone of memory-filled holidays, nightly family dinners, and some of the finest moments with friends. As the mother of daughters, I've wanted to model for them only a healthy relationship with food, ever so watchful that "Mommy writes about weight loss" not translate into body-image issues. Determined to protect them from that type of self-defeating, navel-gazing anxiety, I have never uttered the too-common refrain of women everywhere: "Ugh, I feel fat." So naturally my antennae sprang up when I heard my girls in the backseat of our car.

It began as a simple request for pen and paper. Happy to keep them busy, I told them where they could grab it from a bag I'd packed earlier. Then one asked me, "Mommy, how do you spell olive?" Followed by, "What about chocolate?" "Mommy, can you spell nuts?" I asked them what they were doing, and Sophia replied, "We're making a diet list!"

My blood went cold. I tried to remain calm when I asked them, "For what, girls?"

"Because we're going to go on the Flat Belly Diet!" Olivia announced.

My head began to spin. *My beautiful, perfect babies want to go on a diet? At four?!? What have I done?* Taking a deep breath, I asked, "Um, why?" then steeled myself for an answer like "because I'm fat" or "because my belly's too big."

Then Sophia replied, "Because we want to be healthy!"

Healthy. They wanted to be healthy. We talked a little while longer, and it was pretty clear that the message they'd been hearing me recite during television and radio interviews for months was the one I intended—that the foods on the plan were filled with nutrients that keep you from being sick or tired. And that reaching your ideal weight means you'll have more energy to do the things you love. They'd absorbed the crucial message that is the bedrock of who I am and what I do in my role as an author: Eating wholesome, nutrient-rich food leads to good health, and good health is one key to a happy life.

I share that story with you because it's my mission to help others get the information they need to live better. I want you to be healthy, and I don't want it to be hard. My role as editor-in-chief of *Reader's Digest* provides me with an extraordinary platform to fulfill that mission.

For more than 90 years now, *Reader's Digest* magazine and books have been part of people's homes, families, and daily lives. We've enjoyed that privilege because you, our readers, tell us that each page delivers inspiration, humor, and trustworthy information that both surprises and enlightens you.

If you read *Reader's Digest* magazine, you know that we sort through all the information out there on the subjects you care about most. Then we curate and condense it so that you don't have to.

We've always brought you the best of cutting-edge medical breakthroughs and advances in nutrition, as well as myth-busting and eye-opening health journalism. We sift out the gimmicks and the fads and present the science and the breakthroughs that really work. Often, we make it fun and present information in bite-size nuggets to ensure that it is easily processed. You want actionable insights that you can trust and use immediately.

They'd absorbed the crucial message that is the bedrock of who I am: **Eating wholesome, nutrient-rich food leads to good health.**

That's what I've done with the Digest Diet. I've culled through all the diet hype. I've read the science and watched the trends. I've discovered some new reasons fat creeps on—and tracked down the latest research on how to get it to fade away quickly. With two-thirds of Americans overweight, we couldn't wait any longer to get this information to you. We asked: How can we help solve this problem by doing what we do best? How can we make it easy? The plan here is the answer.

If you picked up this book, you're likely concerned about

your health and unhappy with your weight. Well, we're going to address those things together. The book you hold in your hands is going to kick-start your weight loss in a very real way. And, while it identifies quite a few areas where fat gain is caused by lifestyle and environmental factors, at its heart the Digest Diet is a plan about food: specifically, the healthy, natural foods that have been scientifically proven to shed fat. (You'll read about the specific health-enhancing benefits of individual foods in special boxes called "Digest This.") We've put it all together in a fast, effective plan that will help you drop pounds quickly—and safely.

*Reaching your ideal weight means **you'll have more energy** to do the things you love.*

To prove it, we put 12 men and women with different weight-loss goals on the plan. Their results will astound and inspire you. What you're going to eat—and how you're going to eat it—is going to put you on a path to lower body fat, better health, and improved energy. At the end of our 21 days together, your pants are going to fit better, the scale will make you smile, and your stamina and spirits will soar. Your doctor might even pat you on the back as she sees your health markers improve.

I ask you now to think about what good health means to you. It's important to know what your true goal is before you begin any journey. Good health, to me, is about wringing as much enjoyment out of life as I can each day . . . for as many years as I possibly can. It means being surrounded by family, friends, and work I love. It's about appreciating the body that moves me through each day. Health and happiness go hand in hand. If you've ever had the flu or a bad head cold, you know firsthand that it's hard for you to feel great when your body feels awful; just like it's hard to feel miserable when your body is running on all engines and feeling strong and fit. People say the number one thing they can do to be happier is to get healthier. Guess what? Not only is that true but it also works in reverse: The happier you are, the healthier you will be.

Is it possible to be happy on a diet? Yes. Here you'll discover just how intertwined excess fat and decreased emotional well-being are, as well as how to flip that equation.

Good health, to me, is about **wringing as much enjoyment out of life** as I can each day.

Laugh your way to good health? Yep. Throughout, we've sprinkled humorous stories from our readers to help you keep perspective and give you a chuckle along the way (just look for the smiley faces).

Take care of yourself without guilt? Yes, again. We're not the diet police, just committed to helping you enjoy lifelong good health.

If you choose to begin your journey to better health and happiness by losing weight, this diet is the simplest, safest, and most trustworthy way to get you there. I wouldn't put a diet into anyone's hands if it didn't embody those three elements: simple, safe, and trustworthy.

I wouldn't write it—and *Reader's Digest* wouldn't stand behind it—if the Digest Diet weren't breakthrough, health-promoting, and easy to live by.

And I couldn't bring it home if it couldn't stand up to the most personal test of all: my girls in the backseat of that car.

Chapter

1

"I've been very stressed
and put my children's
needs above my own.
I'm finally ready to
concentrate on myself."
—SABRINA LORENZI,
LOST 9 POUNDS

Fat: The Good, the Bad, and the Unhealthy

The great irony: Successful weight loss comes when you respect your body at any weight and stop demonizing fat.

I **know you're ready to get started.** And I'm excited for you to begin. First, I want to spend a few precious minutes flipping the switch on our attitudes. Attitude toward what? you may ask. Toward fat.

Here's what I mean: I'm not perfect.

I understand that this may come as a shock to nobody, so I'll clarify: I have bulges on either side of my hips that are not attached to anything important, like muscle or bone, and they jiggle when I move. Two scars the size of grapes live proudly on each knee (one from an incident at gymnastic camp when I was a kid, the other from a fall when I was seven months pregnant with my twins). Every evening, I feel the throb of the bunion on my right foot—the one my mother hilariously suggested I might want to remove when I get my "double chin looked at." I have pale freckle-prone skin, thick thighs, bony knees, and a bump on my nose that's evidence of a collision with my then two-year-old daughter.

Yep, that's my body in all its imperfect glory. And I adore it.

Do I sound vain? I hope not. I begin a book about losing weight by telling you that I love my body because *how you feel about yours* is essential to the journey upon which you're about to embark. Finding a place where you are inspired to take care of yourself, but not inspired to beat up on yourself, is crucial to staying on track long-term. Accepting "not perfect" is a great first step.

I've spent the better part of my 20 years in journalism studying health, nutrition, fitness, and the ways that the body does or does not respond to the food we put into it and the movement we ask out of it. As a writer, editor, and author, I've put my body through the most rigorous (and often ridiculous) regimens in an effort to get strong, lean, and fit for myself, as well as to learn what works for others. I've met and mentored thousands of men and women (at book stores, gyms, and sometimes virtually) to both offer encouragement and share a heart-to-heart about the genuine obstacles that can make change hard to achieve. I've been fortunate enough to meet and applaud the many people who've followed my work and succeeded on its advice.

I weigh myself every day (if only because I've found it's easier to focus on *not gaining* weight than living in a cycle of trying to take it off). Over the years, the number on the scale has been as low as 135 (woohoo!) and as high as 173 (yikes!). You may not think that's heavy, just like I may look at you and think the same: What's important is to be comfortable in your skin and to not listen to well-intentioned but wrongheaded people on the subject of your weight. A wardrobe stylist who was dressing me for a television appearance once said to me: "You have a pretty good shape under there. If you lost 20 pounds, you would rock these clothes!"

Did I look in the mirror and imagine what she meant? No.

Finding a place where you are **inspired to take care of yourself** is crucial to staying on track long-term.

continued on page 20

"My Energy Is Soaring!"

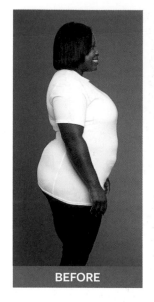

BEFORE

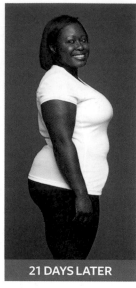

21 DAYS LATER

Adrienne Farr

WEIGHT

BEFORE: **209 pounds**

AFTER: **191 pounds**

TOTAL

18 Pounds Lost!

INCHES

9.5 total inches lost!

3 inches of belly fat lost!

HEALTH GAINS

▶ "I am a lot less anxious."

▶ Reduced back and knee pain

▶ Blood pressure decreased from 128/82 TO 104/68

▶ Reduced total body fat by 6.4%

Adrienne's busy lifestyle as an executive assistant has made it difficult to find the time for healthy habits. But she was ready to change when the scale climbed past 200. Her back and knees hurt, and she was worried about her health: "I knew that my cholesterol was high and my blood pressure (although normal) was creeping higher." A former high school gymnast, Adrienne, 36, yearned to be fit again.

Her first step to success? Healing her mind: "Sadly, even when I was fit and in great shape, I still thought I was fat." Now Adrienne says, "I feel strong and healthy mentally; I want my body to match."

Within days of starting the plan, her energy was soaring. "I literally jumped out of bed at five a.m. I have never done that." She also found that her food tastes naturally shifted. "I craved greens—spinach, broccoli, fennel. That's new for me."

At her first weigh-in, Adrienne lost an amazing seven pounds in four days. "When I saw that happen, I thought,

'Obviously it is working!' Cupcakes, candy, junk food outside my office—I ignored it. I didn't want anything to derail me."

Another big surprise: Bringing more fun into each day helped the pounds melt off. "I loved watching old TV programs—*Rhoda, Good Times, 227, All in the Family, Three's Company*—it made me laugh out loud." To add more movement to each day, she woke up early each morning and danced in her living room.

She enjoys knowing that her success was achieved by doing something grounded in science. "This didn't feel like a fad diet at all. I never thought it was possible to lose so much weight so quickly and in such a healthy way. This is something I can do for the rest of my life."

But most of all, she likes how this way of taking care of herself makes her feel both physically and emotion-ally. "I feel healthy. My skin is glowing, and I don't have headaches anymore! I feel completely optimistic." And five months after the test panel ended, Adrienne is still losing—she's down a total of 50 pounds and counting!

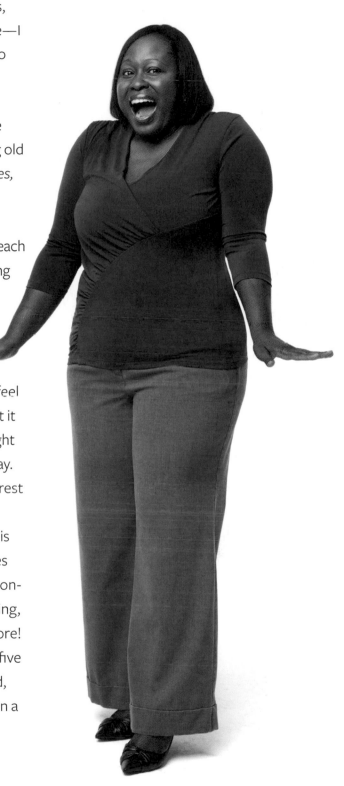

I had a sandwich. And I rocked the outfit anyway. Thing is, I've learned never to look at my own body—or anyone else's for that matter—with disdain. Whether I have 20 extra pounds, too many lumps and bumps, or more aches and pains than I should, I appreciate what God gave me. And I'm here to tell you that this positive mind-set—approaching the amazing miracle that is the human body—is one of the surprising keys to health, happiness, and, ultimately, a shape you'll be proud to live in each day.

There is a subtle but distinct difference between wanting to lose weight and loathing the weight we have. I've met too many dieters who think of their bodies as the enemy. These are the people who won't look at pictures of themselves, who won't go to a beach, who refer to themselves as "disgusting." These are the folks I've watched cycle through an endless loop of deprivation, success, and retreat as they fall back into the self-loathing habits and behaviors that got them into trouble in the first place. It's tragic. It's bad for our bodies and our souls. And it doesn't have to be that way!

If this has been you, that's okay, because I know a secret. It's the secret of successful dieters, and by that I mean the people who lose weight and keep it off. Here it is: These people love and respect their bodies, excess fat and all. They think of their bodies as sacred and worthy of respect, atten-

 LAUGH IT OFF

Following his motivational talk at a Weight Watchers meeting, my father noticed one client's small son climbing onto a scale. "Don't go on that, Joey," warned the boy's slightly older brother. "It makes people cry."   **—CARTER DICKERSON**

tion, and love. It's an attitude—a mind-set—and it works. People who report feelings of aliveness and energy, who, in effect, feel more positive toward life and their daily endeavors, are more successful at staying motivated and at losing weight long-term.[1]

If you're one of those people who need a 'tude up, start here.

● TIME FOR AN ATTITUDE CHANGE

Pause for a moment to think about all the myriad tasks and functions your body performs: It breathes. It digests food. It pumps blood. It loves and learns. It creates the miracle of life. Impressive, right? Yet I've seen people fall into a criticizing rut. My back hurts. I'm tired. My stomach sticks out too much. Somewhere along the way, the body became something to use, mold, shape, and fret about; you don't see its underlying perfection, but instead look for what's wrong with it.

So let me shed some light on why we have fat in the first place, why and where we store it, and how we may have gotten too much of it. It's easier to stop hating something once you get to know it a little better.

● WHY WE HAVE FAT

We were born fat. And that's a good thing. Healthy, full-term babies arrive literally padded in the stuff. Plump, cuddly, and lovely. Scientists theorize that we come packaged this way at birth because newborns need the fat for brain development.

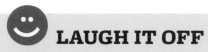

But somewhere along the way, body fat became the enemy, the "lead paint" in your house. The mold in your basement. You want fat gone. You want it gone now.

You might find it strange for me to say this in a diet book, but that type of thinking will set you up to fail. When you think this way, you set the stage to be in a fight with your body rather than an unbreakable, permanent partnership with it. When you regard fat as a foe to be conquered, you're more vulnerable to fall for "quick fix" and extreme eating fads. The human body is meant to have body fat. It couldn't function without it. We even create it so we can store it and use it later, if needed. When you respect that, you'll be more drawn to sustainable, healthy habits.

Why not be creative in how you view body fat and excess weight? Instead of telling yourself that fat is bad, I want you to start a new mantra, one that will release you from an unhealthy belief that will exacerbate any weight issue that might be troubling you:

Body fat is good. You want fat. You need fat.

Yes, you do. (You just don't necessarily want or need as much as you might currently have.) It's our own personal protection against the elements, a builder of cell walls, and our energy storage system, among a whole host of other things explored in this chapter.

● FAT: THE BASICS

Our bodies contain two types of fat: essential fat and non-essential fat, or storage fat. Essential fat is tucked away in our bone marrow, organs, nervous system, and muscles. About 3 percent of a man's body is essential fat; women have a higher percentage, about 12 percent, needed for reproductive purposes. If essential fat gets too low, our bodies won't function properly. That's why it's essential!

Nonessential fat, also known more commonly as subcutaneous fat, plays a few pretty important roles, including insulation against the elements and protection of internal organs. Its other key role is converting excess calories to stored energy. This storage fat, our bodies' energy packs, is nature's way of keeping power at hand (well, often at belly, hips, and thighs) for times of deprivation and shortage. But when this fat gets stored in and around our organs as visceral fat, that's where we run into trouble.

We know now that we need some fat just to function each day. If we get too much of it under our skin? Well, we might not like how it looks, but it doesn't seem to lead to any true health consequences. Deposit too much fat viscerally, however, and potentially deadly health consequences come into play. They include a higher risk of heart disease, dementia, and even certain kinds of cancers.

My aim isn't to scare you. I want to demystify fat, let you know that while it is something that plays many positive roles

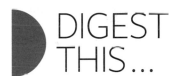

DIGEST THIS...

In one study, people whose diets were **high in trans fats** were more likely to become **depressed** than people who got their fats in healthier forms. This suggests that **olive oil is good for your mood** as well as your heart, while fast food and margarine with trans fats may darken your outlook.

FOUR REASONS TO EAT FAT

While too much of the wrong fat is bad for your health and waistline, a diet rich in the right fat can help both. Here's a quick review of its positive attributes:

▶ **Flavor.** Fat makes the foods we eat taste good.

▶ **Health.** Certain essential fatty acids (EFAs) are only available to us through food, and they're not called essential for nothing. The richest sources of these health-giving EFAs are cold-water fish, nuts and seeds, and leafy green vegetables.

▶ **Energy.** Fat contains the most energy per gram (nine calories). Though it's often cited as a reason to dislike it, a small nibble of healthy fat can sustain your energy for hours.

▶ **Happiness.** The role of omega-3 fatty acids in boosting mood, lessening anxiety, and alleviating depression is well documented.[2] Omega-3s are cardio-protective and potentially cancer-preventive,[3,4] and they are showing promise as a good weight-loss aid as well.

The U.S. government hasn't given a Recommended Daily Intake for fat, but rather a range—20 percent to 35 percent of total daily calories. Aim for that just-right middle place.

The Digest Diet also follows the 2010 Dietary Guideline for Americans: Limit saturated fat to less than 10 percent of our total calories and have a zero-tolerance policy for trans fats, substituting them with a better quality of fats, called polyunsaturated fatty acids and monounsaturated fatty acids (MUFAs and PUFAs).

in our bodies, it can be dangerous. We're all grown-ups. We can take it. So be soothed. Fat is not some mythic monster that you don't stand a chance of slaying. It's there for a reason, and you can safely and healthfully get rid of any excess amounts that endanger your health. Here are a few key points I hope will help you put this overly demonized part of the body in perspective.

Fat Fact #1
Our bodies need fat to live.

Without fat, our bodies wouldn't function properly. Fat is a crucial player in hormone signaling and the creation of reproductive hormones. (We can't reproduce if body fat falls too low, so basically none of us would be alive today without it.) Though our bodies create some fat, certain fats can only be gotten from foods. These essential fatty acids, EFAs, are linoleic and linolenic acid (otherwise known as omega-6 and omega-3 fatty acids). The right balance of these is important to heart health, brain development, mood regulation, blood clotting, and inflammation control.

> About two-thirds of **the brain is comprised of fat,** and it needs fat to thrive and function properly.

Fat Fact #2
Fat protects us.

Fat protects our organs, acting as both an internal cushion and a layer of protection against outside forces. It protects us from the elements, and it plays a key role in regulating and maintaining a just-right body temperature: not too hot or too cold.

Fat Fact #3
We need fat to absorb important vitamins.

We could not absorb vitamins A, K, D, and E without fat—that's why they're known as "fat-soluble vitamins." These vitamins get tucked into our livers and fatty tissue. Though we need only modest amounts of them compared to water-soluble vitamins, they are crucial for healthy eyes, teeth, bones, skin, and cells; infection resistance; and normal blood clotting.

Fat Fact #4
The brain is fat.

If you've ever tasted organ meats, you're probably not surprised to hear that a human brain is mostly fat. About two-thirds of the brain is comprised of the stuff. And, in fact, brain cells rely on dietary fat to synthesize brain and nerve tissue. The bottom line: Your brain needs fat to thrive and function properly.

Fat Fact #5
Fat makes our cell walls strong.

Fat keeps cell membranes resilient and healthy. Two layers of fat actually form cell walls, or membranes, the fortresses that protect our cells. Not only does fat keep the cell frame intact, but it also provides energy for cell function.

Fat Fact #6
Fat *can* make us more attractive.

In our thin-obsessed culture, you might be shocked by the suggestion that fat can make you beautiful. But it's true, and I think it's important to stop demonizing obesity and excess weight . . . to stop assuming that fat has to be equated with ugly. Fat keeps your skin and hair healthy, which enhances your appearance, and if you lose too much of it on your face, you can look gaunt.

● FAT CREEP: HOW DID IT GET THERE?

Whether it's overindulging in too much wine at last night's office party, too many sweets at your husband's birthday bash, or even spending too much time at the gym yesterday (yes, that happens!), you *can* have too much of a good thing. Overindulgence comes with unhappy and sometimes unhealthy consequences, whether it's having a hangover, not fitting into your favorite jeans, or being too sore to stand. And that's also true for body fat.

It's easier than you think for that fat creep to sneak in and make itself comfortable. Likely you were minding your own business, just going along with your life, when suddenly you looked down and were surprised to see a muffin top rolling over your pants or back fat bulging out of your bra. Perhaps you went to your annual physical and saw that big chunky slide on the scale move a whole notch. It's as if you blinked and the weight magically appeared. Seriously. How did *that* happen?

> For most of us, **it's a series of little things.** Small shifts away from self-care, which over time add up to a bigger you.

For most of us, it's a series of little things. Small shifts away from self-care, which over time add up to a bigger you. Maybe it came from moving a little less (your commute

continued on page 30

Slim & No Longer Stressed!

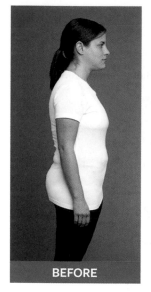

BEFORE

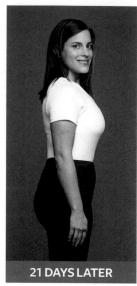

21 DAYS LATER

Christina Ierace

WEIGHT

BEFORE: **145 pounds**

AFTER: **134 pounds**

TOTAL

11 Pounds Lost!

INCHES

7 total inches lost!

2 inches of belly fat lost!

HEALTH GAINS

▶ "My knees don't hurt anymore."

▶ "I have more energy to do more."

▶ Increased optimism and happiness

Christina, 26, is the ultimate multitasker, working a full-time job as a secretary, while also being a full-time student. Burning the candle at both ends definitely has its downsides, though. "I stopped being as active, and my metabolism slowed down. It all just catches up to you. I've only started gaining weight in my twenties; it's been hard." The stress is also affecting her life in other ways. "I can definitely use better sleep. Also, my right knee hurts, and I notice that once I lose weight, it goes away."

All of this motivated her to try again to make a change that would stick. But when she heard about the diet from her aunt, she was a little wary. She'd worked hard on diet after diet, and all ended up disappointing her. "I've tried the no-carb, low-carb, and eating less, but I couldn't handle it because I was so hungry all the time. I am sick of the yo-yo dieting and the minimal and unstable results."

She committed to and followed the diet closely and was pleasantly surprised to find that the foods fit her busy lifestyle. "I really found it easy when it was a shake for dinner," she says, referring to the Fast Release phase. In later stages of the plan, she loved the Big-Batch Roast Chicken (page 173) and what seems to be a team favorite, the Peperonata with Fennel (page 219).

She also found that moving every day was key to sticking with it. She made it a point to walk more, squeezing in 10 minutes here or there and asking friends to join her instead of socializing over meals. "My friends are very supportive and always want to exercise or go bike riding." Some days were harder to exercise than others, but worth it. "When I work out, I don't want to eat junk food because I just worked my butt off."

On the Digest Diet, she's flourished, losing the weight she aimed to shed and discovering a healthy life balance that works for her. One of the first things she plans to do next: give herself a much-needed vacation and revel in her newfound self-confidence. "I just bought a size four skirt yesterday! Instead of saying that I want to go on a diet, I can just say I want to stay the way I am."

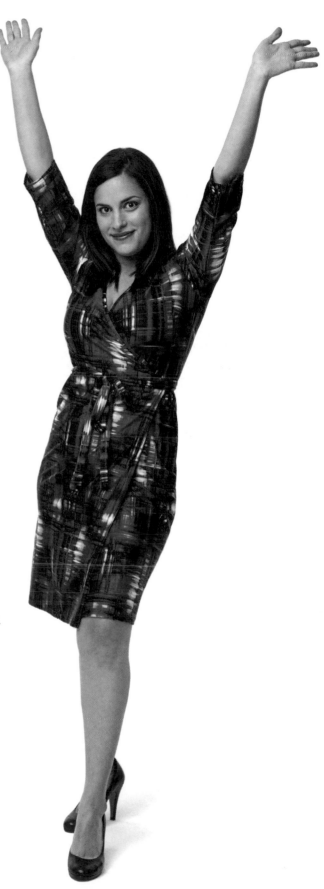

turned from a walk into a car ride). Maybe it came from eating a little more (you began to eat dessert every night instead of once or twice a week; you never checked the calories on your new favorite snack). Or maybe it came from gaining a pound here and there during special occasions or vacations, then never quite taking them off. For women 35 and older, it may have come from a downshift in estrogen production and the resulting uptick in the stress hormone cortisol that often go hand in hand, leading to a deposit in the belly bank. Sigh.

Whatever the scenario, inch by inch, this gradual fat creep snuck up on you. It's time to take charge of the situation, and the Digest Diet is the answer. Just as the fat crept on, we're going to make it just as easily fade away.

● SMOOTH SAILING AHEAD: THE FAT RELEASE DIFFERENCE

Every day, we make choices—some conscious, some not—that can increase fat stores or decrease them. Together, in the coming weeks, we're going to balance the scales. You're going to eat and move in ways that will fill your life with fewer "fat increasers" and more "fat releasers." Many things worked together to cause excess fat to creep onto your body, so you're going to use more than the standard two tools (diet and exercise) to make it disappear. And you're going to use these tools in novel ways. For too long, we've looked at being overweight as simply a calories-in-calories-out equation rather than a whole-body, whole-life experience. That's going to change here.

I've read everything in our database of weight loss and

nutrition research here at *Reader's Digest* and determined what science was credible enough to believe in. Specific foods and behaviors that have been shown consistently to increase the accumulation of fat (or hinder its loss)—I call those "fat increasers." But I've also identified through my review some novel and effective "fat releasers": foods and activities that help your body shed fat more effectively and quickly, to reverse the scale's upward climb. The Digest Diet targets the best-known fat increasers in three key areas—eating, environment, and exercise—and gives you tools to turn the tables on them and go from fat creep to fat release. As added assurance, we tested the plan and its yummy recipes on a panel of people just like you, and you'll hear about their victories and get-real tips within these pages, too. I'm proud of the Digest Diet because not only is it supported by current science, but also it is enjoyable, sustainable, and livable.

In the chapters that follow, you'll get a closer look at the way our eating, environment, and exercise (yes, exercise) can contribute to our growing waists and fat stores. We'll address these big creeps, we'll send them on their way, and we'll have fun doing it. That's right! Laughter and bursts of enjoyment are as central to the success of this plan as the food you put in your mouth.

A healthy, scientifically backed diet plan that helps you shed weight quickly and safely? Plus a lifestyle plan to put energy and laughter back into your everyday life? Who knew releasing fat could be so much fun?

Chapter
2

> "The last four or five years, I couldn't lose weight. The doctor tells me I'm 'middle aging.' I just don't accept that."
>
> —DIANE ROHAN,
> **LOST 11 POUNDS**

Three Fat Increasers

Weight gain is no longer a simple matter of overeating. The subtle reasons Americans are collectively gaining weight will shock you.

Rewind twentysome years to my first job out of college. I was making $7 an hour at a weekly entertainment magazine writing rock music reviews, living with Mom and Dad, and feeling high on life. I didn't have a lot of expenses, and I thought I was generally living within my means. But a funny thing started slowly happening. I bought that cool used leather jacket that would look so amazing on me at the Lenny Kravitz concert. I ordered too-expensive flowers for Mother's Day because that year I wanted to really blow Mom away. I paid for this one dinner, that one theater ticket. I thought, "Just for this one Christmas I'll put some of the gifts on plastic."

Fast-forward five or so years: Lo and behold, I'm looking at a credit card statement and a balance that I'd need to triple my income to ever get my arms around. What an awful feeling. When I got married, I took part of our wedding gift money and paid it all off. I vowed never to carry debt again.

That's exactly what I do with the pounds. I try my best to keep them away so weight loss doesn't become the central focus of my life. This weight-maintenance philosophy has worked well for me for decades. Sure, the scale does occasionally creep up—even a seasoned health editor and diet book author isn't immune to fat creep. But I weigh myself every day so I can quickly and honestly assess what's changed (Am I eating more? Exercising less?) and take action. I know how easily one pound here, two pounds there can multiply and almost overnight become a seemingly insurmountable problem.

It seems like everywhere we turn, something is there that will help make—or keep—us heavier than we should be. I look around and am stunned by the fact that we're literally surrounded by fat increasers. Some are obvious, others not so much. Before I can help you navigate around them, though, we need to understand them, identify them, set them in our targets, then blow them out of the water.

> The **kind of food we eat and when we eat it** can have a major impact on weight loss.

The world can be divided into three areas of fat increasers—potholes, if you will—where we all unintentionally stumble in our quest to keep off or shed some extra padding. They are eating, environment, and exercise.

● FAT INCREASER #1: EATING

Food is a fat increaser. "Well, duh!" you might think. Doesn't take a rocket scientist to tell you that, right? Not so fast. Small variables in our food (the kind we eat, when we eat it, the combinations of food we consume) can have a major impact on weight loss. Did you know that being deficient in certain nutrients can increase your fat stores? Or that when you eat can have a drastic influence on your food choices and your appetite, as well as your risk for disease?

Keep reading. Remember, once you look clearly at what's

affecting your increase in body fat, you can make simple shifts in your everyday choices that will add up to big benefits.

Too Much Food: Fuel, Fakes, and Fads

We've hit the trifecta, folks, but it's a losing hand. Three of the most common fat increasers—fuel, fakes, and fads—are stacking the deck against us. First up: fuel.

No shock here. We take in more food than we use. Researchers in a study published in 2009 in the *American Journal of Clinical Nutrition* found that the increase in food intake alone "appears to be more than sufficient to explain weight gain" in the U.S. population. The estimated difference in daily calories to reverse this is approximately 500 for adults and 350 for children.[1]

Where are we getting all of these extra calories? Are we just pigging out all of the time? Not me. And I'd guess not you, either. Then what's going on? Well, for one thing, we're being faked out.[2]

Food manufacturers want you to buy their products. If you don't, they can't stay in business. To keep their products moving off the shelves, food companies employ food scientists to create new, even tastier versions of foods by manipulating fat, sugar, and salt content. This magic formula makes appealing food even more appealing. And that makes us want to eat more and buy more.

Former FDA commissioner David A. Kessler wrote about this eloquently and shockingly in his wonderful book, *The End of Overeating*. He showed that the balance of fat, sugar, and salt in many of our processed foods literally changes brain chemistry, creating a cycle of addiction. What makes these processed foods even more alluring? They are often time-savers. And the worst thing? These easy-to-use, flavor-rich, processed foods provide plenty of calories, but often, not a lot of nutrition . . . leaving our bodies and our brains literally hungry for more.

I share this revelation not to attack food companies, but to provide a reality check on why it's so hard to maintain a healthy diet in America today. The foods in the Digest Diet are real and wholesome. You don't have to banish all processed foods from your diet forever; the plan utilizes some of the better choices available. But to get back on track, you need to avoid many of the worst offenders for a while.

The Digest Diet doesn't alienate food groups, count carbs, obsess over calories, or surrender to any type of faddish eating behavior (as that, too, has helped add to our collective body-fat increase). The reality is that whole foods, real foods of all sorts, are what your body wants, needs, and should be eating.

CHEW THIS OVER: Check your portions. Don't get all or even most of your nutrition from a box. Think like Mark Twain and remember: moderation and balance.

Not Enough Food: Being Too Strict with Calories

If you read the last section and thought, "That's not me. I am very careful about how much I eat and what I eat. I'm just still more padded than I like," then this one's for you.

Just as too much energy in will lead to fat creation (remember, excess calories get turned into fat and stored as fuel), so can too little. Being too restrictive with your calories can signal to your body that it's time to hang on to what you have.

Our bodies strive for constant and consistent balance, a state called homeostasis. And when that's threatened, they hunker down and hold on . . . and we store more fat as a result.

Think about it: When something threatens your salary or income, your first instinct is to cut back and hang on to the money you have. The body does the same with fat—when the calorie stream it's used to is disrupted, or you start losing the energy stores it has so painstakingly accumulated, the body says: Oh, no. You're not taking this from me!

One study showed that adults **deficient or depleted of vitamin C** may be more resistant to losing fat.

Even worse: If you try to save on calories by skipping breakfast, you're indulging in one of the worst fat increasers. I'm sure this is not the first time you've read how important it is to eat breakfast every day. But do you do it? And do you believe it? If you need further proof of why a morning meal is a must-have, look no further than a 2010 study out of Milan.[3] Researchers found that skipping breakfast leads to increased appetite, poorer food choices, and poor diet quality over all, resulting in a heightened risk of diabetes and cardiovascular disease.

CHEW THIS OVER: Keep your appetite in check—and your waistline—by eating breakfast and balanced daily meals.

Not Enough Micronutrition: Particularly Calcium and Vitamin C

To write this book, the staff of *Reader's Digest* and I read dozens of books, articles, and studies to find the most salient advice to address our unprecedented collective weight gain. One guiding principle we came across again and again: We need to shift the balance of foods we eat so that we embrace more whole foods and more plant-based foods. But why?

At the most basic level: Real food is real good. Really good for you, really tasty, and chock-full of helpful health and weight-loss "buddies" in the form of vitamins, minerals, phytochemicals (substances in plants that help prevent disease), and other micronutrients (nutrients required in small quantities for our bodies to grow and function normally). But exciting research tells us to spend even more time with certain of these buddies if we want to release our extra fat stores.

In 2008, researchers in Quebec, Canada, reviewed a stack of population studies as well as current nutrition research to find what they called unsuspected determinants of obesity. Their review uncovered strong evidence that linked less-than-ideal intake of particular micronutrients to an increased likelihood of being overweight.[4] They identified deficiencies in zinc, magnesium, vitamin E, and vitamin C as risk factors for having a higher percentage of body fat and greater central obesity (that's the unhealthy visceral belly fat mentioned in Chapter 1). More fat and right where we want it least—great!

Calcium is another weight-loss friend cited frequently in studies. Numerous researchers have pointed to how calcium deficiencies are associated with greater fat mass and less appetite control.

continued on page 42

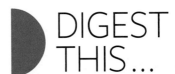

DIGEST THIS...

Here's yet another reason to **eat breakfast!** Choosing the **right kind of carbs** to start your morning can make you double the amount of fat you burn during your subsequent walk or workout, according to a study from the University of Nottingham in England. The key is to **choose carbs that are digested slowly**—that is, unrefined carbs that are high in fiber—instead of ones that your body will burn fast for energy.

Taking Midlife by Storm!

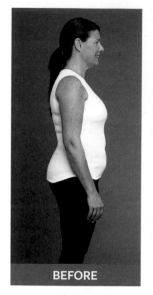

BEFORE

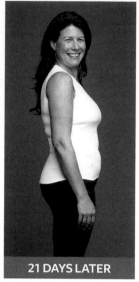

21 DAYS LATER

Diane Rohan

WEIGHT

BEFORE: **185 pounds**

AFTER: **174 pounds**

TOTAL ◀ **11 Pounds Lost!**

INCHES

8.5 total inches lost!

2 inches of belly fat lost!

HEALTH GAINS

▶ "My skin is clear and bright. People ask if I'm getting facials!"

▶ Increased optimism and happiness

▶ Vigorous activities feel easier

"I've been battling my weight all my life. It's like a roller-coaster," says this energetic event planner and mother of a teenage son. She eats well and exercises because it makes her feel good. "I do Zumba. I have a Stairmaster in my house. Working out is what I do for fun."

That's why it's all the more frustrating that since entering her early forties, losing weight has felt like an unwinnable challenge. "The last four or five years, nothing is working. The doctor tells me I'm 'middle-aging.' Well, I just don't accept that, the whole 'You're getting older, you're spreading out, and that's the way it is.'"

The Digest Diet was just the jump start she needed: The 48-year-old experienced incredible results, losing 7 pounds in just four days, and dropping more than 11 pounds in just three weeks.

Around Day 15, she began to experience doubt: The menus provided such a bounty of food, she thought, that she couldn't possibly continue to lose. But the fat releasing menu surprised her and proved its power: "I kept weighing myself in the morning, and the scale just kept getting lower and lower."

She faced another challenge when she joined her family and friends at a local burger joint. "I drank water while people ate burgers and fries. They were laughing at me, saying, 'You're not going to eat anything?' " But she knew she had better choices waiting at home. "I was talking to a friend recently, and we were saying that sometimes you can just say, 'I've had enough of that in my life.' "

She was ready, and she was motivated. "I stuck to this diet. I was determined to lose weight. And I did."

Not only did she succeed in releasing the pounds, she also feels and looks amazing. "I am less sluggish and can zip my size ten jeans!" When asked what's next for her, the answer is simple: "The size eights at the back of my closet!"

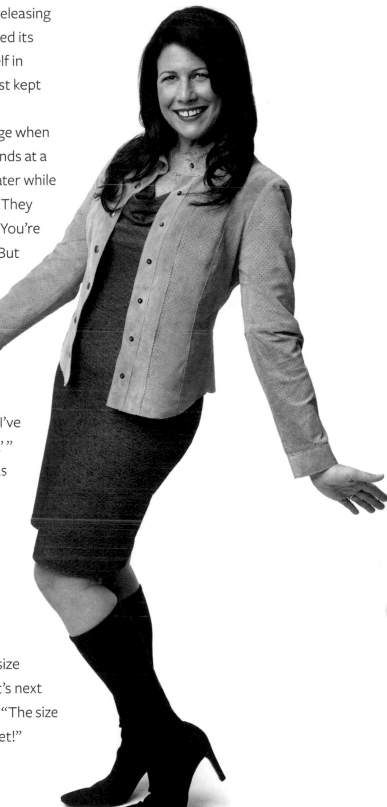

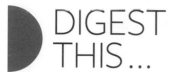

DIGEST THIS …

Is **calcium** the key to a longer life? It just might be, according to a Swedish study. Researchers followed more than 23,000 middle-aged and older men for a decade and found that those who reported getting plenty of calcium in their diets (about 2,000 milligrams per day) **were 25 percent less likely to die** in that time than men who consumed little of the mineral. It's possible that the high-calcium diners had other healthy habits, the researchers say. But a calcium-rich diet can **lower blood pressure, cholesterol, and blood sugar levels.**

Another study showed that adults deficient or depleted of vitamin C may be more resistant to losing fat.[5] And excitingly for us, people who had adequate C levels burned 30 percent more fat during a bout of exercise than those low in C!

Micronutrients may also help us outsmart homeostasis, our bodies' natural desire to hold on to the fat we have. Often, when we start to lose weight, we also start to feel hungrier; we want to eat more. No, you didn't imagine this side effect of weight loss. But how do you get around it? A study published in the *British Journal of Nutrition* in 2008[6] found that micronutrients were key and that people who supplemented with them had less hunger and less of a desire to eat while shedding pounds. On the Digest Diet, instead of reaching for the supplement bottle, over the next 21 days, you will be stocking up on foods rich with these micronutrients.

CHEW THIS OVER: Eat whole foods to lose weight without feeling hungry!

Not Enough Satisfaction

Here is a subtle but key reason that the pounds slowly creep on under our radar: We're not truly satisfied by our food—by what we eat, the way we eat it, and the mind-set we're in when we're eating and snacking. When I say satisfied, I mean two different but equally important things:

There's the physical feeling of being full, satisfied, or satiated from food, and there's the expectation that food will give us emotional satisfaction.

The two are often intertwined. The more we reach for food to make us feel better, the more we get into the habit of soothing our daily stresses with food instead of reaching for other tools. Also, if we allow ourselves to be distracted during our meals—by phone calls, texts, strangers ringing the doorbell, the television, or too many tasks—our feelings of satiety can be disrupted. That's why infusing more joy into each day and focusing on staying present in each moment—and at every meal—is a fundamental must-do on this plan.

CHEW THIS OVER: Eat foods that trigger fullness (we'll show you how). Do one thing at a time. Fill up with friends, fun, and laughter.

● FAT INCREASER #2: ENVIRONMENT

Hands up! You're surrounded . . . by fat increasers, that is. Not only do you have to navigate through the minefield of overabundant fake foods that surround us all, but each day, you have to try to skip over landmines you may not even know exist. Some of these hidden fat bombs include chairs, beds, and even the air we breathe.

As you already know, eating certainly plays a part, but our daily living environment is also a prominent factor that sets the stage for fat accumulation.

Too Many Chairs

We would all throw our chairs out the window if James A. Levine, M.D., of the Mayo Clinic had his way. Dr. Levine is

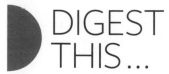

DIGEST THIS...

If you work or play at the computer while eating, **your waistline may suffer.** In a recent study, volunteers who played a computer game as they had lunch ate **twice as many cookies** a short time later as people who didn't multitask during their meal.

the affable and incredibly smart researcher who has spent years looking into some pretty NEAT things (Non-Exercise Activity Thermogenesis). NEAT accounts for the calories we burn through the activities of daily living—all the ways we move that aren't formal exercise. It's what we use up by doing spontaneous physical activity (SPA): bending, sitting, walking, fidgeting, combing our hair, hugging our children or spouse, doing a favorite hobby, or cooking dinner. Obviously, we burn more by living a full life rather than by sitting on our bums and watching it go by.

Why should we care about such small moves? Because we're not getting enough of them, and it's clear from the collective state of our waistlines. On average, SPA can lead to a calorie burn of about 348 calories each day—as many as 700 calories a day for the more fidgety among us. That's a chunk of calorie-burning love. Especially when you take into account the daily 500-calorie shift researchers estimate stands between us and a healthy weight. It also explains how SPA protects against fat-mass gain.[7]

CHEW THIS OVER: Don't sit still. This is one place where you definitely should not listen to your mom.

Too Much Thinking

If your job includes physical labor, you're likely moving quite a bit each day and getting a NEAT benefit from it. But if you're like many office workers, you get a double whammy: Not only are you sitting at a desk for most of the day, but this type of mental, knowledge-based work actually makes it more difficult to control appetite and may make us eat more calories and fat.[8]

Research suggests that because brain neurons rely almost exclusively on glucose as fuel, intense mental work leads to unstable glucose levels. Since the work requires glucose for maximum brainpower—well, we naturally reach for more fuel.

CHEW THIS OVER: The Digest Diet relies on hunger-fighting foods to help outwit your appetite while working.

Too Little Sleep

How long you sleep directly affects your body mass. Whether you snooze too much or too little, it's not good for your health or your waistline. Too much and you're at higher risk of becoming overweight. Too little and you plant the seeds that blossom into weight gain: Sleep deprivation interferes with the hormones leptin and ghrelin that regulate our appetite. That means you'll feel hungrier and are more likely to indulge in poorer eating behaviors. Also, you may look for more "energy" in the form of unhealthy snacks!

All lead down the same unhappy path to increased weight. But it's a little bumpier

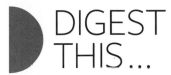

DIGEST THIS...

If vegging out in front of a TV is your favorite hobby, you may be courting an early death—even if you're not overweight. That's what Australian researchers found after tracking nearly 9,000 people for an average of six years. Regardless of their weight, **those who watched television** for more than four hours daily had a **46 percent higher risk** of death, compared with people who channel surfed for less than two hours. (Americans watch TV for about five hours each day.) Television itself isn't the problem, says study author David Dunstan, Ph.D., of the Baker IDI Heart and Diabetes Institute. Instead, the **danger comes from all that sitting**, which takes the place of activity.

for undersleepers because the hormonal changes lead them to store fat in the abdominal region.[9]

CHEW THIS OVER: Try to sleep seven to eight hours a night—you'll have more energy and reduce cravings.

Too Much Pollution

The rigorous readers on my editorial staff keep bringing the research to my attention: The toxins, chemicals, and compounds riddling our food supply and self-care products are contributing to the nation's collective fat creep. Study after study shows that organochlorine compounds, specifically, adversely affect the body's ability to oxidize fat—they resist being metabolized and are readily stored in fatty tissue. These compounds have been found in plastics, herbicides, and pesticides, as well as chlorine-based household products.

Other fat-inducing toxins literally surround you. Did you know that the very air you breathe, if you're eating a high-fat diet, might actually induce insulin resistance?[10] A study done in 2011 at the College of Public Health at Ohio State University found just that: Exposure to fine particulate matter (air pollution) induced insulin resistance, reduced glucose tolerance, and increased inflammation, leading researchers to mark long-term exposure to air pollution as a risk factor for diabetes. And as we know, diabetes and obesity are close cousins (80 to 85

LAUGH IT OFF

After noticing how trim my husband had become, a friend asked me how I had persuaded him to diet. It was then that I shared my dark secret: "I put our teenage son's shorts in his underwear drawer."

—RUTH J. LUHRS

percent of those diagnosed with Type 2 diabetes are obese).[11]

CHEW THIS OVER: Reduce your exposure to the toxic soup that surrounds us. Choose organic when it's convenient and affordable. Buy a good-quality air filter, if you can. Your health and waistline will thank you for it.

Too Little Joy

I'm sure you could make a laundry list of all the things that cut into your personal good cheer each day. But how often are you truly playful? Just being a grown-up frequently means that responsibility takes the driver's seat, while being silly and spontaneous gets thrown in the trunk. Adulthood is a serious ride.

You don't need a researcher to tell you about the link between stress and obesity. It's pretty clear-cut: Many of us self-medicate with food when we're feeling blue, anxious, or depressed. But what you might not know is that heightened anxiety can lead to the greatest of double whammies—more fat and an increase in belly fat accumulation.

And these fat cells don't just affect your waistline: They can actually increase your risk of depression. According to Drew Ramsey, M.D., a psychiatrist and coauthor of *The Happiness Diet*, "Fat cells are metabolically active, meaning they send signals

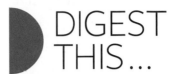

DIGEST THIS...

Want even more reason to get some Zzzs? Check out these study results:

- 4.7 percent of adults reported **nodding off** while driving in the past 30 days.

- Sleep-deprived people often **consume an extra 300 calories** a day.

- Sleeping less than 6 hours per night can increase **your risk of developing diabetes by 30 percent** by impairing your body's ability to regulate blood sugar.

- **Here's a zinger:** Dieters who got 8½ hours of sleep nightly lost 56 percent more body fat than they did when eating the same diet but getting just 5½ hours of sleep a night.

Still think you don't need to get your 8 hours straight?

to brain cells and, as such, affect brain function. We know that being obese greatly increases the odds of being diagnosed with a mood disorder like depression or an anxiety disorder. For many, this may stem from the chronic low-grade inflammation that can be tracked back to fat cells."

Just one more reason it's important to stop fat creep before it affects your emotional health and well-being.

CHEW THIS OVER: Get down on the floor and play with a kid, settle in to watch the comedian or comedy show that makes you laugh the hardest, stand outside and watch the sunset. Look for little ways each day to fill yourself with more joy and less stress.

● FAT INCREASER #3: EXERCISE

If you're scratching your head wondering how it's possible that exercise could possibly be a fat increaser, stick with me. In no way am I suggesting that exercise is bad for you. On the contrary, the list of reasons to get your daily move on is so long that it could fill an entire book.

But exercise on its own (when it's isolated from a healthy eating plan) is not a great weight-loss agent.[12] It does make for a pretty great preventer of weight gain, though. And

 LAUGH IT OFF

Although I was only a few pounds overweight, my wife was harping on me to diet. One evening, we took a brisk walk downtown, and I surprised her by jumping over a parking meter, leapfrog-style. Pleased with myself, I said, "How many fat men do you know who can do that?"

"One," she retorted.

—R. T. MCLAURY

the good news is that a quality plan can help push aside fat creep, especially when combined with the right fat releasing diet. But the wrong kind of exercise can make you eat more than you intend.

Same Old, Same Old

Nod your head if you do the same workout over and over. You just hit that treadmill, elliptical, or jogging path and you put in your time. Time after time. You feel like you're challenging yourself; you really do. But if you're honest, there's a certain sameness to your routine.

When the research started coming out in the late 1990s, I was shocked to learn that focusing solely on continuous cardio might actually have been contributing to the pound a year I gained during that time. (*Seriously?* I hear you say. Yes, seriously.) Aerobic exercise (the kind that makes your heart pound and your body sweat) demands that you increase your energy output. Because our body is always trying to stay in balance, this type of movement may actually act as a biological cue to make you eat more. Researchers also believe that cardio may cue additional eating because it depletes glycogen stores in the liver and muscle in order to make glucose available for fuel.[13]

Besides making you eat more, continuous aerobic exercise isn't nearly as effective a weight-control strategy as surprising your body with aerobic interval training (short bursts of high-intensity, heart-pounding work) or strength training (push-ups, squats, anything that builds muscle and power).

The Fat Release Workout (page 246) combines both—strength and high-intensity interval training (HIIT)—into a 12-minute workout that's amazingly effective for fat burn and muscle growth. Don't worry. It will be fun (and brief!).

CHEW THIS OVER: The smartest fat-loss exercise strategy is to work hard in short bursts and mix it up!

Thinking You Are Working Harder Than You Are

I've seen a lot of research in my day, but this one really shocked me. How you look at the exercise you do affects whether or not you'll keep lost weight off. Those who perceive that they are working very hard, even when they aren't, are more likely to regain weight.[14]

One 2010 study noted that women who self-reported feelings of low vitality and poor emotional health over-perceived their efforts during exercise.[15] Feeling blue and blah led them to believe they had worked out harder than they had. It's obvious how this misperception can lead to weight gain; if you truly think you're working it hard when in reality you're sitting this one out, the pounds will absolutely find a way to creep on to you.

CHEW THIS OVER: Keep a log of the time you spend moving each day; write out exactly what you did for exercise. It may surprise you.

Relying on Exercise Alone to Control Weight

From 1998 to 2006, I was the executive editor of *Fitness* magazine. Studying the fitness research and trying the trends were all part of my job. For years, I believed that I could eat anything I wanted because I was exercising so much. I was spending nine or more hours a week running, walking, biking, lifting weights, crunching my abs, relaxing and stretching my limbs in yoga, doing Pilates, and more. I exercised like a fiend. And I ate like a linebacker. But I'm here to tell you, the more I exercised, the hungrier I was. And the more I ate, the more I needed to exercise to maintain a healthy weight. Here's what happened: I saw a steady increase in my body weight of a pound a year.

Thinking you can eat whatever you want as long as you work it off later is actually a pretty dangerous mind-set, particularly if you look at the current research. Exercise alone leads to a very modest decrease in total body weight: less than 3 percent![16] (Scarf down a pint of ice cream and you'll be running a *long* time to work off the fat and calories. . . . Marathon, anyone?)

The good news here is that exercise reduces visceral fat, the dangerous kind, independent of whether you lose weight.

CHEW THIS OVER: To be effective as a weight-loss agent, you have to pair exercise with the right diet—this one.

Going to the Gym

If we actually went there, this wouldn't be on the list. But often, we just don't get around to hitting the gym. We are too tired. Too busy. Too stressed. We're always too something. And as a result, it's one of the first things to not do on our to-do list.

Don't hamstring what you can accomplish each day by making your exercise dependent on going somewhere to do it. The

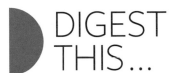

DIGEST THIS...

We know that **exercise is a great stress reducer,** and nowhere is this more important than in **battling cancer.** Among women with breast cancer, those who did yoga had a **steeper daily drop in levels of the stress hormone cortisol** than women who just stretched.

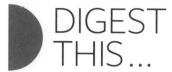

DIGEST THIS...

only exception is if it's an activity you absolutely adore; if you love doing something, its location becomes irrelevant.

All of the moves in the Digest Diet Fat Release Workout are designed so that you can do them at home or around your home, without equipment. Just you, the floor, a chair or a couch, and a towel or a mat.

CHEW THIS OVER: You don't have to exercise hours and hours a week to lose weight. Move a little every day, and match it with the right eating plan.

Choosing Exercise You Hate

Many people don't like to exercise. I'm not one of them, but that doesn't mean I was always this way. I made a conscious choice on my thirtieth birthday that fitness was going to be part of my daily life—no excuses, no sabbaticals, no dreading it. I understand that formal exercise is not fun for some people and never will be. And I also understand that asking you to do something you dislike intensely will only stand in the way of long-term weight control.

I want you to do the exercise portion of this book because it will make you stronger and it will give you a great fitness foundation. But at the end of the 21 days, I want you to work very hard to find something active that you like. Whether it's walking through the park or riding a bike with your kids. The only must is that you must enjoy it. The research is on your side on this one: A study by Swedish researchers looked into the attitudes, strategies, and behaviors important to weight maintenance. One of the significant strategies successful maintainers employed? They'd found the joy.[17]

This gels completely with the work of Barbara L. Fredrickson, Ph.D., author of *Positivity*, Kenan Distinguished Professor, and Director of the Positive Emotions and Psychophysiology (PEP) Lab at the University of North Carolina at Chapel Hill. This leading scholar graciously shared the following with us: "Our research shows that if a new wellness behavior evokes positive emotions, people are 4.5 times more likely to be continuing with that new behavior 15 months down the road, enjoying all of its healthy benefits. It appears that positivity is the key to lasting lifestyle change. Enjoyment motivates sustained change by creating nonconscious desires that are far stronger than conscious willpower. It's best to select ways of eating and being physically active that you truly enjoy. Those are the only lifestyle changes you stand a chance of getting 'hooked' on, and that's what's needed for long-term weight-loss success."

CHEW THIS OVER: You gotta love it!

I hope by now you're saying, "Wow, I had no idea that so many fat increasers are affecting my habits, appetite, weight, and happiness." Believe me, once I saw how all this evidence stacked up, I understood why fat creep has affected me and is such a common complaint among both male and female readers.

Now I can help you take control. In the next chapter, you're going to learn about the key elements of success on the Digest Diet. They are the fat releasers—the simple foods and behaviors that will make the fat fade away.

Chapter 3

"My new 'Cafe Mocha': a cup of coffee with two teaspoons unsweetened cocoa and two teaspoons honey. It's full of fat burners."

—STAN GNIAZDOWSKI, **LOST 16 POUNDS**

Three Fat Releasers

Frustration-free weight loss equals joyful living: Nourish yourself with real food, find ways to move and play, and laugh a little every day.

I remember poring over the astonishing research on MUFAs (monounsaturated fatty acids) for *Flat Belly Diet!* and feeling so excited that I had stumbled upon a nutrient that helped the body shed fat. I feel the same way now as I learn about the fat releasing properties of vitamin C, calcium and dairy, protein, and more.

It thrills me to be able to assure people that weight loss is not a hopeless push-the-boulder-up-the-hill effort that you have to return to again and again throughout your life. The solutions are within your reach! They are in the very foods that probably fill your shopping cart every week. They are in the easy choices you make each morning when you roll out of bed! They are as simple as making a shake, having a laugh, even sipping a glass of milk.

In fact, certain foods, actions, and activities can gently shift your body into fat release mode. Some will be intuitive after reading Chapter 2, in that you can choose to do the opposite of what led to fat increase; others will require a plan of attack so that you can gracefully skirt over these landmines.

The 21-Day Fat Release Plan (see Chapter 4) is built around adding as many fat releasers to your day as is achievable, practical, and enjoyable. Ironically, the fat releasers I'm about to tell you about are very similar to the fat increasers: eating, environment, and exercise. What that means: Tiny shifts in your habits in these three areas can reverse the scale's upward climb.

● EATING: FOODS THAT RELEASE FAT

The Digest Diet calls on a rich, diverse array of foods to help you get back to your desired weight. But who doesn't want a shortcut for accomplishing it, when possible? Why take the long way when you can go straight to where you need to go?

I'm all about getting the most out of every moment of your day—and that means choosing foods that give you the most out of every bite. The Digest Diet makes foods that can actually amp up your weight loss the staples of your diet in a way that's easy and delicious. So that's the focus here: discovering the ideal choices to have at hand to keep you satisfied, your calorie burn set to its maximum output, and your energy levels soaring.

Fat Releaser #1
Vitamin C

You've heard for years to stock up on your C when you're feeling a cold coming on, but until you opened this

 LAUGH IT OFF

Although I knew I had put on a few pounds, I didn't consider myself overweight until the day I decided to clean my refrigerator. I sat on a chair in front of the appliance and reached in to wipe the back wall.

While I was in this position, my teenage son came into the kitchen.

"Hi, Mom," he said. "Whatcha doin', having lunch?"

I started my diet that day.

—BETTY STROHM

book, had you ever heard of it as a fat-loss aid? As mentioned in Chapter 2, suboptimal levels of certain micronutrients will undermine your efforts to maintain a lean body and avoid belly fat. Folks with inadequate C levels? Well, their bodies seem to cling tight to fat.[1]

CHEW THIS OVER: According to the most recent DRI (dietary reference intake) tables put out by the National Academy of Sciences' Food and Nutrition Board, the recommended daily allowance for this important micronutrient is as follows: Women should aim for 75 milligrams a day; men, 90 milligrams daily.

Fat Releaser #2
CALCIUM

Your mom told you to drink milk because its calcium was good for your bones. But I doubt she knew that the calcium in it was also great for controlling hunger. Remember the discussion of suboptimal nutrition? Research shows that those who have deficiencies in calcium hold a greater fat mass and experience less control of their appetite— two things you can reverse on this plan.

CHEW THIS OVER: The DRI for calcium is as follows: Women under age 50 should aim to take in 1,000 milligrams of calcium each day; if you are older than 50, that number should shift upward to 1,200 milligrams daily. Men, throughout adulthood, should aim for 1,000 milligrams of calcium daily and when past the age of 70, up that to 1,200 milligrams.

◗ DIGEST THIS…

The mineral **potassium** can cut your **risk of stroke** by more than 20 percent. Sweet potatoes and tomato paste are the most concentrated sources of potassium; bananas and **low-fat dairy foods are good, too.** If you're on an ACE (angiotensin converting enzyme) inhibitor or other blood pressure medicine, though, be sure to **talk with your doctor first;** you may want to avoid potassium-rich foods.

Fat Releaser #3
DAIRY

This fat releaser may sound like a repeat of the last, as dairy is an excellent source of calcium. But, even more excitingly, studies have found that dairy sources of calcium are markedly more effective in accelerating fat loss than other sources,[2] so I've separated it out as a fat releaser. Researchers theorize that other ingredients in dairy act synergistically with the calcium. I love the two-for-one nature of this fat releaser!

I found even more exciting research suggesting how to use dairy to maximize your fat fading results. In one study out of the University of Tennessee, researchers showed that eating three servings of dairy daily significantly reduced body fat in obese subjects. If they restricted calories a bit while continuing with the same dairy servings, it accelerated fat and weight loss.[3]

There's more! I found a great study done in 2010 that showed that drinking fat-free milk immediately after whole-body resistance training and then one hour after the workout resulted in "greater muscle mass accretion, strength gains, fat mass loss, and a possible reduction in bone turnover in women."[4] Drink milk and increase fat loss, strengthen bones, and gain more strength and muscle? Sign me up!

CHEW THIS OVER: Eat at least three servings of fat-free or low-fat dairy each day. Time it with your exercise so that you can maximize milk's effectiveness.

Fat Releaser #4
PROTEIN

I love this macronutrient powerhouse for so many reasons, including that it promotes healthy skin, hair, nails, bones, and muscle. Protein exists within every cell in our bodies, and it influences everything from enzyme and hormone production to wound and tissue healing. But my two favorite benefits for the purposes of the Digest Diet? Well, they were shared in a 2005 study out of Arizona State University that looked at proven strategies for successful weight loss. Researchers found that protein increased satiety (satisfaction and feelings of fullness) and increased after-meal thermogenesis (this is a fancy word for calorie burn).[5] Eating protein as compared to higher-carbohydrate meals leads to more satisfaction, less hunger, and more fat burn. I love that: Three benefits in one!

Drink milk and increase fat loss, strengthen bone, and build muscle? Sign me up!

Earlier research found that people following higher-protein diets generally decrease their food intake by an average of 10 percent (about 200 calories). Eat protein and naturally eat less? Great!

CHEW THIS OVER: The RDA for protein for women is 46 grams daily; for men, 56 grams. Can you eat more than this healthfully? Yes, which you'll see and enjoy in Fade Away, the second phase of the Digest Diet.

Fat Releasers #5 and #6
PUFAs and MUFAs

Those of you who've read my earlier books know that I am solidly behind foods rich in monounsaturated fatty acids, or MUFAs. Eating a diet rich in olives, olive oil, nuts and seeds, dark chocolate, and avocado has kept my belly flat and my energy up for years! These healthy fats are a mainstay of my diet and an essential part of this plan as well.

But in my dive into the current research, I came across a study from the Netherlands that suggests we better not forget to enjoy another group of fatty acids—polyunsaturates, or PUFAs—found in fish and its oil and in many nuts and seeds, including peanuts, walnuts, sunflower seeds, flaxseeds, and sesame seeds. Subjects in this study showed that consumption of PUFAs lead to a higher RMR, resting metabolic rate (the calories used just to live), as well as a greater DIT, or diet-induced calorie burn.[6, 7] PUFAs are also burned faster than saturated fats in the body. Another win-win for us.

But one clarification: Our focus will be primarily on long-chain n-3 PUFAs, more commonly known as omega-3s. As mentioned earlier, some of the amazing health benefits of omega-3s range from cardiovascular protection to mood enhancement. So why would these fats reduce body fat? Researchers theorize that the weight-loss benefits of omega-3s result from their anti-inflammatory effects[8] (inflammation in the body has been strongly linked to obesity).

Our diets generally have more than enough of another kind of PUFA: n-6, or omega-6s. So focus your attention on balancing the scales on the side of the weight-loss-friendly and mega-health-promoting omega-3s.

CHEW THIS OVER: Women should aim for 1.1 grams of omega-3s daily, men 1.6 grams.

Fat Releaser #7
COCONUT OIL

While we do limit the amount of saturated fats eaten on the Digest Diet, one fat sits at the top of the "should enjoy" list: coconut oil. Why? This sweet, rich oil was shown to do some pretty nifty things for abdominally obese women

continued on page 64

Breaking a Plateau at Age 52!

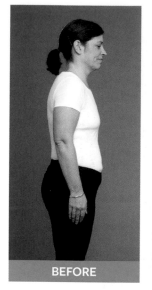

BEFORE

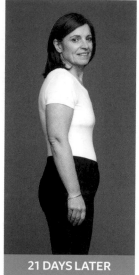

21 DAYS LATER

Annette Procida

WEIGHT

BEFORE: **165 pounds**

AFTER: **154 pounds**

11 Pounds Lost!

TOTAL

INCHES

Almost 6 total inches lost!

1.5 inches of belly fat lost!

HEALTH GAINS

▶ Lost 4.8 percent of total body fat

▶ Everyday activities feel easier

This busy working mom of three had come to a full stop. After losing 50 pounds, her weight loss had come to a standstill. She needed a jump start. "I've been on a successful weight-loss journey for two years, but I hit a brick wall."

She believed that the plateau was due to the hormonal changes going on in her body. "My weight was up and down, and I couldn't break it. So many people have told me that when you hit menopause, you stop losing weight—I won't let that happen. I felt that this diet came at the right time, to help me put my body back in losing mode."

Boy, did she do just that, losing 11 pounds in three weeks. According to Annette, "I didn't have a hard time. In the beginning, I was a little freaked out when I saw those shakes and soups. I thought I would be starving. But to tell you the truth, that was my favorite part! It was filling; it was delicious; it was easy." (Her fave shake flavor: apple, peanut butter, and cinnamon.)

One major factor in Annette's success: her 23-year-old daughter,

Dana, who did the Digest Diet with her mother and lost 8 pounds in three weeks. They had each other's backs the whole way: Dana packed their lunches and snacks, while Annette cooked for the two of them in the evening. Says Dana: "We enjoyed making the recipes together, putting love into the food."

What else added to their success? They both exercised every day. "That is what I enjoy and take the time to do for myself," says Annette. "My mom inspires me to take care of myself," adds Dana.

Annette intends to reach her goal weight of 145 pounds by continuing with the Digest Diet (and she plans to do it with her other daughter as well). She urges others to try it. "This way of eating can be done every day without any problems. Just go with it. You're going to enjoy every single thing you eat." And her advice to those who fall off the path is simple: "Sure, you are going to want to eat something you love, like pizza or pasta, but that's okay. You have a guide to get right back and keep on going with your new, healthy way of eating."

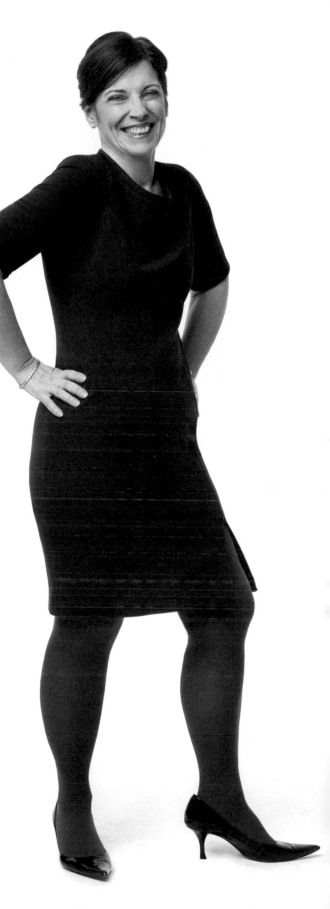

in a 2009 study out of Brazil, including decreasing their waist circumference (belly fat), increasing beneficial HDL (high-density lipoprotein) cholesterol, and improving the ratio of "bad" LDL (low-density lipoprotein) to "good" HDL cholesterol.[9] Also, in populations where coconut oil is commonly eaten, high cholesterol levels and heart disease are not common.[10]

> **CHEW THIS OVER:** We tend to consume more than our share of saturated fats, so we're going with the RDA here: Limit saturated fat content to 10 percent of your total calorie intake each day, and make coconut oil or coconut milk one of your top sat-fat picks.

Fat Releaser #8
RESVERATROL

So many people have asked me if it's okay to have a drink when trying to lose weight. Listen up, friends, as this glass is for you!

Many studies have been done throughout the years that clearly show that a small glass of wine a day is good for your health. Now numerous animal studies are highlighting its great promise as a fat releaser. The resveratrol in red wine (found in red grapes, mulberries, and peanuts, too) has antiaging researchers racing to see who can unlock the fountain of youth first. While they busy themselves with that, we can benefit from the cutting-edge research that suggests this antioxidant is a fat releaser.

> In one study of middle-aged women, **those who drank moderately had less weight gain** than those who abstained.

In one large study of more than 19,000 middle-aged women of normal weight, those who were light to moderate drinkers had less weight gain and less risk of becoming overweight than those who drank no alcohol.[11] In several animal studies, researchers have demonstrated that moderate alcohol consumption does not promote weight gain.[12] And in another separate animal study done in 2006, the researchers found that resveratrol improved exercise endurance as well as protected against diet-induced obesity and insulin resistance, a precursor to diabetes.[13]

> **CHEW THIS OVER:** A four-ounce glass of red wine each day won't hurt your weight-loss efforts ... in fact, it may help!

Fat Releasers #9 and #10
FIBER AND VINEGAR

Throughout the years, various weight-loss researchers have recommended starting a meal with a salad to stave off hunger and ensure that you don't overeat. But why does this work, exactly? One reason is that salads are a great source of fiber: lettuce greens, carrots, tomatoes, and the like all have plenty of this macronutrient. Fiber is absolutely your friend when it comes to feeling full; its effects on increasing feelings of satiety are well documented. So the Digest Diet is chock-full of it—and don't worry, we get plenty of fiber from things other than salad, if you're not a fan of it!

Another substance that often comes along for the ride in a salad is vinegar. Research has shown that vinegar can reduce the blood-sugar spiking effect of a meal, which has been linked to satiety, resulting in reduced food intake. You feel more satisfied, you eat less. But vinegar may also prevent body-fat accumulation, according to an animal study done by Japanese researchers in 2009. In that study, mice were fed acetic acid, the main component of vinegar, for six weeks; this suppressed the accumulation of body fat in the animals.[14] Whether you eat them together or not, know that fiber and vinegar are great tools to have on hand whenever you feel the need to tame your appetite and turn on fat-burning controls to cruise into the best shape of your life.

CHEW THIS OVER: There is no RDA for vinegar, but it certainly can't hurt to have it each day in your favorite salad dressing or in another recipe. As to fiber needs: Women under the age of 50 should aim to eat at least 25 grams each day; if you are over 50, try for at least 21 grams. Men have higher fiber needs. If under age 50, you should consume 38 grams each day; 31 grams if over 50.

Fat Releasers #11, #12, and #13
QUINOA, HONEY, AND COCOA

The Daily Fat Release Menus (see pages 122–142) utilize these three fat releasers regularly, but in moderation; honey and cocoa, if overused, can add unneeded excess calories to your diet. What do the three have in common? All may lead to less fat deposition in our bodies. Nibble on the information below to learn a little more.

Quinoa. I'm keen on quinoa for a number of reasons: This ancient grain is a nutritional powerhouse, chock-full of protein, amino acids, phytosterols, and vitamin E. We should all be eating it just for its nutrition profile alone!

A study published in 2011 points to its

DIGEST THIS…

A study of 2,471 men and postmenopausal women found that those who consumed **one to two glasses of beer or wine daily** had up to 8 percent denser bones than teetotalers. And red wine is chock-full of resveratrol, which, in addition to its role as a fat releaser, has been shown to **protect against bone loss** in animal studies. Don't go overboard, of course. Excess alcohol can actually harm bones, and too many calories, if you drink too much, will hinder your weight-loss efforts.

promise as a fat inhibitor. Animals supplemented with an extract made from quinoa seeds showed less body fat, decreased body weight, and decreased food consumption.[15]

Honey. Similar to quinoa, honey has also shown great promise in animal studies for reducing weight gain and adiposity (fatness) when substituted for sugar.[16] It's a nutritious alternative, and its health properties are wide-ranging: It has antibacterial, antiviral, and antifungal properties. It may improve blood sugar control, is a great cough suppressant, and it improves immunity.[17]

Cocoa. If you're like me, you welcome any new excuse to add more chocolate to your life. Cocoa contains more antioxidants than most foods and is good for so many things. Just look at this benefits list from a recent study done at the Yale University Prevention Research Center by David L. Katz, M.D., and his colleagues: "Cocoa can protect nerves from injury and inflammation, protect the skin from oxidative damage from UV radiation . . . and have beneficial effects on satiety, cognitive function, and mood."[18]

In an article published in the June 2011 edition of the *Journal of Nutrition*, researchers looked at the effect that epicatechins, a substance found in cocoa, had on obese diabetic mice. (Since a diabetic's lifespan is, on average, seven years shorter, they were looking for any antiaging promise that increasing dietary intake of this flavonoid might give.) Their findings: The mice lived longer. The cocoa reduced degeneration of their aortic arteries, and it blunted fat deposition.[19]

CHEW THIS OVER: Enjoy these three whole foods regularly and stop that fat creep in its tracks. Try the Creamy Quinoa breakfast cereal on page 159 for a fat releasing triple-threat treat!

● ENVIRONMENT: BEHAVIORS THAT RELEASE FAT

Next up: simple things you can do to shift your lifestyle and your perspective so the fat stops creeping on and starts fading away.

Fat Releaser #14
FIDGET IT OFF

If too little NEAT and SPA (see page 48) leads to excess weight, then finding ways to build more modest movement into your life is one key to reversing it. Some folks just naturally move more than others. They fidget, twist their hair, scratch their faces, get up and down every few minutes. (My girls never seem to stop moving!) We now know from research at the Mayo Clinic that those who are naturally lean (you know the sort: They seem to eat all day, whatever they want, and never gain a pound or an inch) automatically, even subconsciously, find ways to move to make up for any extra calories they may be ingesting. That's just biology. And it differs in all of us. Some of us just like to sit, ponder, and stay put. But that's one way the pounds will also stay put. So what can you do if you're not a natural-born mover? Consciously make choices that naturally boost your burn without breaking a sweat.

> Make choices that **naturally boost your calorie burn** without breaking a sweat.

Don't phone it in. When making or taking a phone call, stand up and pace a bit. Do this each time you pick up the phone and it will really add up.

Be the remote. Whenever you have to switch a channel, instead of sitting and surfing, stand up and walk over to the

TV to do so. You might be saying, I have no idea how to change a channel without the remote. That's okay: I just want you to get in the habit of standing up for your health here.

Be the dishwasher. Not only will you save water and electricity, it's one way to soak up some calories.

Get comfortable with inconvenience. Look at the common devices in your life that are meant to give you convenience (often meaning that they save you from moving, which isn't saving us at all). How can you use them differently, or not at all, to add a little NEAT? Chop veggies by hand, not in a food processor. Hand-wash your car rather than take it in for someone else to do. The choices are endless.

Step away from the desk. Every hour, no matter how busy you are, make it a point to get up from your seat and walk around your office or home. Even better: Take two laps around the interior or exterior.

Think on your feet. Set up your office or workspace so that you are required to get up and move to accomplish some of your daily tasks. Walk around while texting or e-mailing, rather than sitting at a desk to do so. (Warning: Don't do this while walking up and down stairs, and definitely not outside while crossing streets!) Go visit a colleague, rather than e-mailing them. James A. Levine, M.D., in his book *Move a Little, Lose a Lot,* even recommends people conduct

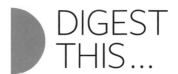

DIGEST THIS...

We all know that **too much sitting is bad** for our hearts—but how much can it help to pop up now and then for a trip to the watercooler? A lot, research shows: **People who took plenty of short breaks** (even if they lasted just a minute) **had smaller waists** and lower levels of a protein that signals potentially dangerous inflammation.

walking meetings. It can't hurt to see if you can interest your employer, colleagues, or employees in doing this.

CHEW THIS OVER: Lots of little moves add up to a big difference—to your health and to keeping you at your healthiest weight.

Fat Releaser #15
SNACK IT OFF

Whether you're at home or go to an office each day, one of the fastest ways to derail your efforts is to not be prepared to healthfully satisfy your hunger when it strikes. And snacking is one of the first areas where we frequently get off track. The key is to surround yourself, and bring with you when traveling or working, nutrient-dense and calorie-poor snacks. All the snacks in the 21-Day Daily Fat Release Menus (Chapter 5) have been designed to incorporate at least three satiety-inducing fat releasers: fiber, vitamin C, and dairy or calcium. They also all have a combination of textures, so that your mouth is satisfied with the crunch and the creaminess . . . and you won't have to grab for potato chips, candy bars, ice cream, or other calorie-loaded, nutrient-poor choices.

CHEW THIS OVER: Don't wait until hunger strikes to find whatever snack you can most quickly lay your hands on. Plan instead for a snack attack and carry your own, so that the pounds won't sneak in, but nutrition will! Enjoy any of the ideas in the Daily Fat Release Menus, beginning on page 122, and you can't go wrong.

Fat Releaser #16
SLEEP IT OFF

If you have trouble getting to sleep or getting enough sleep, you're in good and significant company. Whole books have been written on the topic, so you don't need me to do so here. You know from Chapter 2 that getting fewer than seven to eight hours of sleep each night will increase belly fat and heighten cortisol levels. So we need to flip this equation so that sleep is working for you, not against you. From now on, your nighttime focus will be to shore up on your sleep.

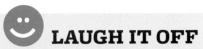

LAUGH IT OFF

My sisters and I have weight problems and are always sharing diet tips. One day, my oldest sister was showing us a low-fat cookbook and pointed out a chicken dish that she had tried the night before. Reading the ingredients, I commented, "It looks like it would taste really bland."

"It did," she replied, "until I added cheese and sour cream." —A *READER'S DIGEST* READER

Though I can't make you go to sleep, I can give you a few tips on getting to sleep that have worked for me and others in the past.

Go to bed earlier. When you're overtired, an unhappy cycle can get started where you can't fall asleep, so you stay up (and maybe you watch or read or do household chores ... or eat) until your body finally gives in. Then you wake up and overcaffeinate, sugar up, and start the cycle all over again. Push the stop button on this unhealthy spin by going to bed earlier, before you get your second wind or, worse, get hyper-tired. Experiment with the time by ending your day earlier, by a half hour or 15 minutes at a time. See what works best for you so that you rest easier.

Just breathe. Sit comfortably in your bed and spend five minutes just paying attention to your breathing. Nothing else. If your to-do list wants to jump in and disrupt you, no worries; just mentally push it all away and go back to focusing on your breathing. Practice this regularly and you'll be sleeping like a baby in no time (and getting a whole slew of other health benefits that meditators worldwide enjoy!).

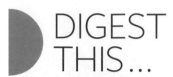

DIGEST THIS...

Did you know that **cardio workouts may help with asthma?** We first announced this in *Reader's Digest* magazine, but it's worth repeating: Aerobic workouts cut asthma symptoms **in people with moderate or severe forms of the disease.** And as is true with your health in general, you should talk to your doctor before beginning any diet or exercise plan.

Grab a scientific journal or textbook. Raid your kid's backpack for his math text or find a dull and dry guide to bricklaying. Whatever you choose, it has to be a snooze. Pop it open and give yourself 10 minutes to read it. Then snap off the lights. A bored brain will likely decide it would rather sleep than read one more word!

Know your ABCs. A friend recently told me about this method she learned at a sleep clinic years ago. It works like a charm. Visualize yourself individually tracing each letter of the alphabet with a pencil, then taking a big eraser and, reversing the path you just mentally drew, erasing each as you progress along the alphabet. I never get past L.

CHEW THIS OVER: If you have tried everything and sleep is still a serious issue for you, don't go it alone. Talk to your doctor. She can help you figure out a plan that is best for you.

Fat Releaser #17
CLEAN IT UP (AND OFF!)

This might be the shortest section in the book, as only you can decide what fits your lifestyle and your wallet: Go organic and avoid toxins wherever you can, whenever you can. If that means you buy organic versions of your five favorite fruits and veggies—or you fill your entire cart with them—it's all good. If it can mean buying a HEPA-grade medical air filter for your home, it's also good. Any choice you make that eliminates toxic chemicals in your life is health-affirming. (And it can be cheaper sometimes, particularly when it comes to household cleaning products. Baking soda, lemon, olive oil, vinegar are all effective nontoxic cleaners—and you can cook with them, too!)

Fat Releaser #18
LAUGH IT OFF (EVERY DAY!)

Stress takes an enormous toll on your health, waist, and immunity. And, as *Reader's Digest* has said for nearly a century: Laughter is the best medicine. But did you know that laughter actually burns calories? Fun, huh? I found a novel study, commissioned by the comedy channel GOLD (Go On Laugh Daily) in Great Britain, where a research team led by Helen Pilcher, Ph.D., formerly of London's Institute of Psychiatry, looked into the number of calories burned by intense laughing and compared it to the calorie burn of other daily activities (strength training, running, even vacuuming). The results of the GOLD study? They found that intense laughter in and of itself can give you a bite-size cardio workout: An hour of it can burn as much as a half hour hitting it hard at the gym! Laughing burns calories, but it can also boost total energy expenditure by up to 20 percent. To put that into perspective: One hour

 LAUGH IT OFF

I was talking to my doctor about a weight-loss patch I had seen advertised. Supposedly you stick it on, and the pounds melt away.

"Does it work?" I asked.

"Sure," he said, "if you put it over your mouth." —MARY KAAPKE

of laughter burns up to 120 calories, about the same as 18 to 27 minutes of weight training, 15 to 20 minutes of walking, or 40 minutes' vacuuming.

CHEW THIS OVER: Watch your favorite sitcom and burn calories? What a hoot!

● EXERCISE: MOVES THAT RELEASE FAT

Remember how your approach to exercise—mentally and physically—can lead to unintentional fat creep? Now we'll focus on the strongest methods for using exercise to accomplish your weight-loss goals. Have fitness work with you, not against you, as you fade the fat away.

As you now know, it's important to get more nonexercise movement into each and every day, and one great way to do that is to walk. But to really maximize your calorie burn and release those pesky fat stores, you have to turn to strength training and aerobic interval training. In Chapter 7, you'll find our simple workout that combines all of these elements so you fight fat creep and increase fat loss with a 1-2-3 punch. But first I want to explain why strength training and working hard in short bursts, or intervals, is the most efficient use of your time and energy—and drives the fastest results in terms of calorie burn and fat loss.

Fat Releaser #19
LIFT IT OFF

My aim is to save you time and to save your sanity while you try to fight the fat that's parked itself in places you don't want it. And one of the best tools in your fitness bucket is

OUR TWO-FOR-ONE WORKOUT

The beauty of the Fat Release Workout in Chapter 7 is that it combines two powerful fat releasers—strength training and HIIT—into one easy 12-minute routine. The strength-training moves are designed as intervals that will have your heart pumping, so you get in the aerobic benefits of HIIT at the same time as you build muscle. HIIT is thought to be effective because of the mix of intense effort and recovery time within an aerobic workout; our regimen on page 246 mimics that effect within a simple, straightforward strength routine. Remember, what's important is intertwining effort and rest, to keep your body guessing and the fat releasing.

Normally, this type of training requires a fairly high level of fitness, but this workout is designed so that anyone can do the routine, regardless of fitness level, and all can be done from the comfort of your own home and without any equipment. Start there and soon enough, you might be "bursting" your way to the best shape of your life.

Besides the fat burn and improved cardiovascular conditioning you get from interval training, you also get another bonus—intense bouts of exercise actually lower the hunger hormone ghrelin.[20] You can maximize this side effect by starting the day with a morning workout.

high-intensity strength training. This doesn't mean an hour at the gym every day. Nope, not unless that's what gives you joy. Instead, research out of the Department of Kinesiology at Southern Illinois University showed that as little as three 11-minute intense strength-training sessions a week resulted in an increase in fat burn at rest and a chronic increase in energy expenditure throughout the day. In short, it increased resting metabolic rate as well as calories burned during sleep![21] How's that for a liftoff?

CHEW THIS OVER: The more muscle you have, the more fat you burn.

Fat Releaser #20
HIIT IT OFF

A growing body of research suggests that bursts of intense activity mixed in with rest time is the fat releasing, muscle-building, power-promoting way to go for weight loss—and it's great for your heart.[22]

As mentioned in Chapter 2, aerobic interval training in the form of HIIT (high-intensity interval training) is a great way to power off the fat creep, and it's best to do so in short workouts. What's involved? Basically, if you're doing HIIT in the traditional way, you want to warm up for about 4 minutes, then go hard at your fastest pace through your favorite cardio (a 30-second row, stationary bike, elliptical, treadmill, or stair-stepper "sprint"). Then actively rest for 30 seconds. That means slow down to a snail's pace to catch your breath. Then do it again. Repeat this sequence six times. Take another 2 minutes to gradually power down, with shorter bursts and longer recovery times, and you're done. That's it. A 12-minute workout. You can extend it if you like, but it's best to keep it to no longer than 16 minutes in total from warm-up to cooldown. If you're new to interval training, 12 minutes will be more than enough!

CHEW THIS OVER: The intervals—when your body doesn't know what to expect next—are what give this training such fat releasing power. See our two-for-one workout (box, opposite) to learn how to get the benefits of HIIT and strength training in one easy 12-minute routine.

Fat Releaser #21
LOVE IT OFF

What makes you happy? What gives you joy? What ways of moving and fitness excite you the most? Do you like to go solo and challenge yourself to marathons, runs, and swimming laps? Or maybe you like something slower and sweeter, like walks, nature hikes, and gardening? Do you love to dance? Golf? Or are team sports your thing? Baseball, soccer, football, foosball (hey, if you're standing and moving, it counts!)? If you're saying none of the above, what do you like? Wii? Rollerblading? Biking? What takes you back to the freedom and fun of childhood and puts a smile on your face?

It doesn't matter what it is that makes you want to move. Just be sure that whatever it is, you love it enough to want to do it more.

CHEW THIS OVER: You thought you'd *like* to lose it? Nope. You have to *love* to lose it!

Now that we've explored the common fat increasers and fat releasers, it's time to put it all together in a plan that will stop fat creep in its tracks: The 21-Day Fat Release Plan!

Chapter

4

"I used to inhale four double cheeseburgers in two minutes. Now I'm satisfied with a 35-calorie piece of cheese."

—JOE RINALDI,
LOST 26 POUNDS

21-Day Fat Release Plan

The delicious, natural foods that make weight loss easier—and the simple rules for eating them.

I hope you're as excited to start our plan as I am to share it with you. It's fast, fun, and effective. As you've seen throughout the book, our testers are living, breathing proof that the Digest Diet can change your body—even your life. I can't wait to hear from you after you've scored the winning "fatdown" at the end of the next three weeks.

In this chapter, you'll find the general rules by which to live, eat, and move each day. (The following chapters give you specific menus, delicious recipes, and fitness moves.) I want you to have an overview of each of the tools at your disposal before you begin. Then you can just dive right in and fade the fat away.

After covering the basics, we'll go through the specifics of the food plan itself, detailing what you can expect from each of the three stages, as well as the unique features each brings into the mix. I'll also give you a comprehensive list of the top fat releasing foods. Every meal, snack, recipe, dessert, and menu item on the plan has been crafted to include these satisfying, health-promoting, delicious foods.

By the way, if you heard "rules" and thought, Oh, boy, here comes another confusing, constricting list of must-dos, don't worry. Consider these "rules" information nuggets—small tactics to call on during any stage of the diet. Keep them handy—if it helps you to do so—as you progress through the plan. After, they'll offer inspiration, information, and some practical ideas on what to do if you find yourself stumped. Reach for them whenever you need them. They're meant to be an anchor, not to anchor you down.

● RULES TO LIVE BY

Rule #1: Laugh Daily

You must set aside a minimum of 30 minutes each day to laugh. Preferably, this will mean spending time with someone with whom you usually share a good chuckle. But in our busy lives, that may not be possible to accomplish daily. So think about what makes you laugh loudest, then go for it. For some, that might mean DVRing a favorite sitcom or watching Comedy Central; for others, it might mean taking a time-out during your busy day to go to a humor website. (One of my favorite ways: flipping through this book to find the Laugh It Off sidebars!) Whatever it means to you, you must take the time to do it!

 LAUGH IT OFF

Needing to shed a few pounds, my husband and I went on a diet that had specific recipes for each meal of the day. I followed the instructions closely, dividing the finished recipe in half for our individual plates. We felt terrific and thought the diet was wonderful—we never felt hungry!

But when we realized we were gaining weight, not losing it, I checked the recipes again. There, in fine print, was "Serves 6." —**BARBARA CURRIE**

Rule #2: Rethink Convenience

Over the next three weeks, look closely at your life and the conveniences (read: fat increasers) around you. What things can you do differently each day to add in more fresh food? How can you add in more movement? Can you get up to stretch, bend, or walk? Can you garden inside or out? Been longing for a dog? Nothing says fat burn better than three or four extra walks with Fido each day.

Test Team FAQ

I have a headache, and I feel like I might be coming down with a cold, as my sinuses are clogged. Could the diet be causing this?

Liz: Have you stopped drinking caffeinated beverages? That's a well-known cause of headaches. If you're a caffeine drinker, enjoy a cup a day of the caffeinated beverage of your choice. But no soda! Also, are you drinking enough water? Make sure you're drinking water throughout the day and staying hydrated. If your body is used to a lot of processed foods and sugars, it's possible that you could be experiencing symptoms like that of a detox diet because you've made this healthy switch. None of our testers had these feelings last more than a day or two.

Rule #3: Sleep

You know how good a good night's sleep makes you feel. Now you know that it's also a cozy and enjoyable way to release fat. Do whatever it takes so that you can snooze to lose.

Rule #4: Remember the Middle Place

In all that you do, the best way to succeed, be healthy, or be happy long-term is to aim for that middle place where moderation, balance, and good sense are the rules of the day.

Rule #5: Don't Go It Alone

Our testers found that having group support through a Facebook page we set up was incredibly useful for staying on track

HOW TO EAT AND EXERCISE AT-A-GLANCE

▶ Eat breakfast.

▶ Eat real food. Choose whole foods over processed. When you need to use packaged products—and we all do— choose those with an ingredients list that's no more than five items (or as close to it as possible).

▶ Go organic whenever you can. Whatever you can do is a step toward health. Just do your best.

▶ Choose fat releasers at every meal and snack (our daily menus make it easy).

▶ Thrive with five: Look for fiber, protein, vitamin C, calcium, and dairy in your food choices.

▶ Eat three servings of fat-free or reduced-fat dairy each day.

▶ Exercise first thing in the morning.

▶ Exercise hard in short bursts.

▶ Mix up your moves to keep your body guessing.

▶ Remember, if you can make exercise fun, the battle has been won.

and inspired. Surround yourself, whether it's online or with your best buddy on the phone, with people who will support your efforts. (Go to readersdigest.com/digestdiet or facebook.com/digestdiet to get tools and encouragement from *Reader's Digest* and your fellow Digest Diet participants.)

THE 21-DAY FAT RELEASE PLAN

FAST RELEASE: Days 1 through 4

FADE AWAY: Days 5 through 14

FINISH STRONG: Days 15 through 21

The eating plan is organized in three basic stages: Fast Release, Fade Away, and Finish Strong. Every phase loads you up on fat releasers. But the calorie and macronutrient ratios shift to maximize weight loss—and results!

Fast Release is a four-day fat releasing jump start. During it, you're going to shed fat quickly and safely (our biggest loser on the test panel lost 10 pounds in four days!). This phase is about flooding your body with nutrition with a diet rich in soups and shakes. And we've found solid science behind why fast, early weight loss is important to long-term success.

Fade Away transitions you into lean proteins and micronutrient-rich greens. For this 10-day stretch, you continue to have a shake a day, but the lean-and-green focus gives your body what it needs to help you release fat and build muscle, while lowering your intake of carbohydrates for faster fat fade. If you like, enjoy a glass of red wine with dinner. If you're not a drinker, red grapes are a sweet substitute.

Finish Strong is the last week of the plan. The meals and recipes show you how to enjoy a balanced, whole-foods

> ## Test Team FAQ
>
> I'm not a great fan of drinking milk. Can I add cocoa to make it taste better?
>
> **Liz:** Yes. You can add cocoa powder, but remember that the Digest Diet recommends unsweetened cocoa powder. Try ½ teaspoon. If you still don't care for the chocolate milk, you can eat an equal serving of nonfat yogurt in place of drinking milk.

diet rich in fat releasers. If you haven't reached your goal at the end of three weeks and you want to shed more, this is where you stay until you've done so. It's also perfectly fine to cycle through Fade Away and Finish Strong until you reach a healthy place. The Finish Strong phase is a great model for weight maintenance as well, teaching you how to eyeball proper portions and eat a healthy balance of carbs, protein, and fat.

Fast Release: Days 1 through 4

Fast Release focuses on amping up nutrition while giving you speedy results. Why is it important to lose fat fast? Well, besides giving you a great psychological boost right out of the gate, it may also help you keep the weight off longer. A 2010 study out of the University of Florida, called TOURS, demonstrated that shedding weight fast leads to larger overall weight loss and longer-term success in keeping it off. In this study, Lisa Nackers and her colleagues analyzed data collected on 262 middle-aged women. To those of us who are used to hearing that slow and steady wins the race, their results were a little shocking and counterintuitive. The authors' conclusion: "[W]ithin the context of lifestyle treatment, losing weight at a fast initial rate leads to greater short-term weight reductions, does not result in increased susceptibility to weight regain, and is associated with larger weight losses and overall long-term success in weight management."

FAST RELEASE

▶ Drink two shakes a day as meals

▶ Eat one crunchy snack a day

▶ Have soup for one of your meals

▶ Drink plenty of water each day; sip throughout the day between meals and snacks

Drink Two Shakes

A variety of delicious shakes are going to be your weight-loss partners throughout the next two weeks. During Fast Release, you'll be "shaking off" the pounds with two of these nutritive blends each day. The menu plans have been designed so that you start the day off with a shake. When you drink the other is entirely up to you—lunch or dinner. It's a matter of your tastes, needs, and preferences.

Snack Once a Day

You must snack between meals on the Digest Diet, particularly during Fast Release, as calories are slimmest during this stage. I've found that snacking on foods that are crunchy is often the most satisfying way to stave off hunger between meals. Also, since you'll be "drinking" so much of your nutrition through shakes and soups, I wanted you to have the satisfaction of sinking your teeth into something with a little more chew.

You will have one snack a day during the first four days, then two snacks a day during the course of the rest of the plan. Make them at home and carry them with you. Each snack on the menu plan contains vitamin C, fiber for crunch and satisfaction, and protein. For the best results, follow the menus as written (they've been carefully balanced for portions as well as micro- and

DIGEST THIS...

Chocolate milkshakes are a fun part of the Digest Diet. So you'll be delighted to hear that in a study first published in *Reader's Digest* magazine, it was shown that volunteers who ate 3.5 ounces of **dark chocolate** (the gourmet kind that's 70 percent cacao) every day for a week **raised their "good" HDL cholesterol** by 9 percent. That's a load of chocolate (about 550 calories' worth!), but study coauthor Paul A. Gurbel, M.D., of Sinai Hospital in Baltimore, says eating smaller daily doses (say, ½ ounce) over an extended period of time should also help.

macronutrients). But it's also more than okay to choose your favorites to have on hand at your desk, the gym, or wherever your travels take you.

Soup It Up

The word "soup" doesn't do our recipes justice. I can't wait for you to try some of these fiber and protein power-houses! Each one is intended to fill you up with these two fat releasers, while making sure you have plenty to share (or to store for later). The plans have been crafted so that these big, warm, flavorful, comforting bowls are your lunchtime meal. But you can choose to eat soup at supper. Only you know your own hunger hot spots—those spans in the day when you need energy most or feel the hungriest and only something warm and hearty will do. If you find a favorite soup, don't be afraid to switch it for another on the plan. The recipes make nice big batches, so enjoy your favorite as often as you like. Again, follow your own tastes and food preferences, but be sure to stick to two bowls a day during Fast Release.

> Our soup recipes are intended to **fill you up with fat releasers,** while making sure you have plenty to share!

Drink Plenty of Water

Even though you're getting a good deal of liquids from shakes and soups in Phase 1 of the plan, it's still important to stay hydrated and sip plenty of water between meals. Often, feeling hungry or tired is a sign of dehydration, so getting enough water by day is just as important as getting enough sleep at night. Proper hydration can also help you adjust to the healthy journey you're undertaking—some of

continued on page 90

A Family Man Gets Healthy

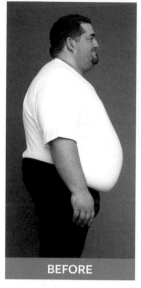

BEFORE

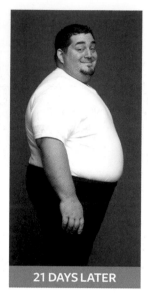

21 DAYS LATER

Joe Rinaldi

WEIGHT

BEFORE: **394 pounds**

AFTER: **368 pounds**

26 Pounds Lost!

TOTAL

INCHES

7.75 total inches lost!

2 inches of belly fat lost!

HEALTH GAINS

▶ Less knee pain

▶ Easier breathing when walking up stairs

▶ "I feel in control of my eating."

Even though he's always been active, Joe Rinaldi has been struggling with his weight for some time. "I have been on diets all my life. I have counted points, done Nutrisystem, LA Weight Loss . . . You name it, I tried it." They worked for a while, and then the weight would return.

Over the past two years, the weight began to seriously interfere with his life. He struggled to ice skate with his four children, one of their favorite ways to have fun together. "It's hard to tie my skates and get my equipment on. I'm in tons of pain. I have to take breaks. I'd like to chase them all down instead of sitting down."

So he was highly motivated to try again. "I don't know what you can lose in twenty-one days, but it will be a good start," he said before Day 1. Well, he lost 26 pounds in three weeks! Not just a good start, but a great one!

His wife and several coworkers did the diet with him, and the group support kept him on track. "Having people checking in on me and pulling for me has kept me one hundred percent on it." But at this point, Joe's motivation comes from within. "I honestly love the diet. If you follow it, it really works. I even set my parents up with it." Another key factor was discovering that he could enjoy healthy food. "After those first days of soups and shakes, I was actually craving good food."

He admits that the first days on the diet were challenging. "But once I got over that hump, it was smooth sailing. As we started eating more, my cravings went away. I never thought twenty pistachios would hold me, but they did." He also made sure to add some fun into each day by playing with his daughters and doing puzzles.

After three short weeks, he finds it easier to breathe when he's walking up steps, and his right knee feels less pain. But that's not all. "I have more energy. I feel like I have control of my eating. I even feel more confident at work. My clothes fit better, and I'm looking forward to taking the rest of my weight off. I feel like I am out of the rut I was in."

At this pace, he'll be skating rings around his youngsters in no time.

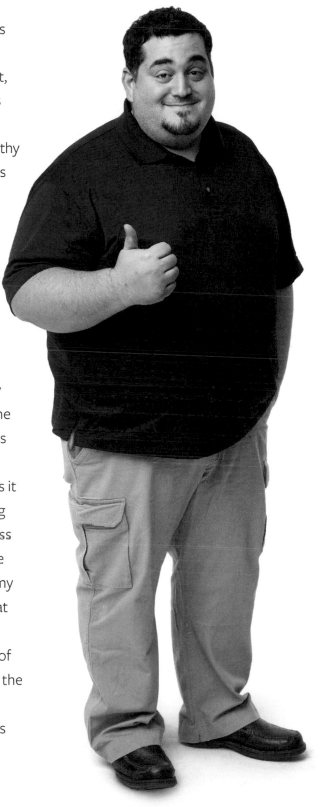

our test panelists noticed that they felt headaches come on when they didn't remember to drink up.

Fade Away: Days 5 through 14

Go lean and green. That's the theme of the next 10 days. While a little lower in carbohydrates than the others, this stage is replete with healthy fats, lean meats, and reduced-fat cheeses, as well as a bounty of vegetables.

You'll probably feel a little like you've taken a trip to Greece or Italy during this stage. And that's a good thing in more than one way. A Mediterranean-style diet is one of the healthiest ones around, and you'll even be enjoying a glass of wine or a bunch of delicious red grapes with dinner. Both are good sources of one of my favorite fat releasers: resveratrol.

FADE AWAY

▶ Drink first, eat second

▶ Have one shake a day

▶ Go lean (proteins) and green (veggies) at meals

▶ Choose MUFAs and omega-3 PUFAs for your healthy fats

▶ Snack twice a day

▶ Enjoy a glass of red wine or a bunch of red grapes at dinner

Drink First, Eat Second

Have a big glass of water with a quarter to half a lemon, lime, or orange before each snack and meal. Not only will you be getting a nice bump of vitamin C and needed daily hydration, you'll also get another bonus: a natural acidic curb to your appetite.

Drink One Shake

Remember, the menus are flexible. I like the shake as a breakfast meal because they're such a rich source of calcium and dairy. That means they're a smart choice before or after the 12-minute workout. Their two fat releasers mean they can maximize the fat fading impact of the exercise. If it's a strength-training day, have it an hour after your workout.

After four days of shakes, I wanted to start mixing things up a bit for you. You'll see we've added in some other protein-rich breakfast options to the menus. My favorite: Creamy Quinoa, with five fat releasers!

Go Lean and Green; Pair with MUFAs and PUFAs

The key to this stage is to fill up on lean protein and vegetables. It's a snap with the lunches and dinners that are simple to prepare. Tasty meals and health-promoting foods—neither has to be tricky!

Our menus have us cruising to the Mediterranean with gifts from the land and sea (chicken, eggs, beef, pork, and fish) as well as a smorgasbord of vegetables (from broccoli, garlic, spinach, and cauliflower to kale, tomatoes, and peppers). In keeping with your desire to incorporate the healthiest fats you can into each day, prepare these foods only with extra-virgin olive oil and other healthy MUFAs and omega-3–rich PUFAs.

Snack Twice a Day

Here's the snack rule for this phase: Reach for protein, fiber, and C. Choose hard-boiled eggs and slices of turkey, chicken, and other lean meats. Enjoy

Test Team FAQ

One of the healthy fat options in the shake recipes is raw almond butter. It costs $14 a jar! Is it okay to skip this ingredient and just stick to the other options?

Liz: Of course! The raw almond butter is there to give you healthy variety, but regular almond butter and natural peanut butter are great (and cheaper) alternatives. That's why we tried to give you so many options in the shakes—so you can customize them to your taste and budget.

fat-free and reduced-fat cheeses, sunflower seeds, almonds, peanuts, or peanut butter. There are a slew of choices on the menu from which you can pick, and they are controlled for calories, too, so stick to our suggested portions.

Drink a Glass of Red Wine

If you don't drink alcohol, other foods can provide you with resveratrol, including a juicy bunch of red grapes. So have them instead. But if you're like many of our readers who have wondered whether wine and weight loss could go hand in hand, you can happily enjoy a meal with a nice guilt-free glass of red. If you're a woman, stick to four ounces (a small highball glassful). Men can have six ounces.

Finish Strong: Days 15 through 21

By this point in the plan, you should be looking and feeling pretty great. Now's the time to hone your focus on fully living the notion of balance that is so integral a part of the Digest Diet. That means training yourself to think in terms of balancing your protein, fat, and carbohydrates. It means filling your plate with a wide variety of fat releasers while remembering to thrive with five (see page 83). It means making sure to take time each day to enjoy your life, enjoy yourself, and slide in some fun. Remember, on this plan I expect you to be actively searching for fun each day so that food isn't getting subbed in for living. No

FINISH STRONG
▶ Bring a balanced eye
▶ Continue to drink first, eat second
▶ Continue to snack twice a day
▶ Continue to enjoy a glass of red wine with dinner
▶ Enjoy a dessert or favorite treat once a week

matter how busy you are, no matter what curveballs life throws you, taking the time each day to find even a little joy is crucial.

Bring a Balanced Eye

In this stage, you'll see an even wider variety of foods on the menu: from sammies and wraps to whole-grain pastas and scrumptious pizzas. Remember, on the Digest Diet, we enjoy good food and aren't interested in eliminating any categories of them; the only exception is trans fats . . . they are never on the menu! With everything else, remember to balance your plate with a variety of foods and a mix of fat releasers. The menu plans and recipes are all properly portioned, so the balancing is done for you in this stage. Pay attention this week. This is your portion-control practice period for real life, the time to learn what amounts to put on your plate and what going overboard looks like.

Continue to Drink First, Eat Second

Often we confuse hunger with thirst. One way around it is to drink a large glass of water before meals and snacks. Not only will it take up some space in your stomach, you'll also be keeping your

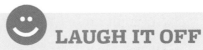

LAUGH IT OFF

The biggest loser at my weight-loss club was an elderly woman.

"How'd you do it?" we asked.

"Easy," she said. "Every night, I take my teeth out at six o'clock."

—CATHY J. SCHREIMA

Test Team FAQ

Where do I find flaxseed meal?

Liz: Most supermarkets and all natural food stores carry flaxseed meal. Look in the aisle where you get your grains, or ask the store clerk. If your store doesn't carry it, go online to bobsredmill.com. Another option is Hodgson Mill, at hodgsonmill.com.

body hydrated. This way, you'll be better able to gauge real hunger.

Continue to Snack Twice a Day

Now fruit is included in your snacks in addition to the tried-and-true fat releasers.

Continue to Enjoy a Glass of Red Wine

Raise a glass to yourself for being in the final stretch of the diet! You are definitely toastworthy.

Enjoy a Dessert or Favorite Treat

Having fruit as dessert each night once you are through with the plan, though, is perfectly acceptable. As for decadence, let's think of that as a once-weekly treat.

Now that we know the basics of the eating plan, let's take a look at the delicious variety of fat releasing foods that you'll be eating and what to put in your cart at the supermarket.

😊 LAUGH IT OFF

Mother and I were discussing our mutual weight problem one evening, when I challenged her to a contest. If I lost the most weight in the next month, I wouldn't have to pay her the $6 that I owed her. If she lost the most weight, I would have to pay up. Anything for an incentive!

"All right," said Mother happily, "but let's wait two weeks before we start. There are some things I have to eat first."

—IRENE LANE

● THE FAT RELEASER FOOD LISTS

Here, I've listed the foods that are the top sources of the various fat releasing nutrients discussed in Chapter 3. As you'll see, these are delicious, nutrient-dense, wholesome foods. No scary diet foods here! As you continue to eat in the way we suggest on the Digest Diet, you'll notice many other foods contain the elements identified as fat releasing. Not to worry. This only means that, lifelong, you'll have a delicious time choosing among them.

For the purposes of these lists, we chose foods for each category that were the best sources of that particular fat releaser or had good amounts of multiple fat releasers, so that every bite would be to your fat fading benefit.

When a food has multiple fat releasing nutrients, it's grouped within the category where it has the most of a micro- or macronutrient. That means if it's a source of fiber and C but it's richer in C than fiber, you'll find it listed with the C foods. What if it's a close call and the food is strong in two or more fat releasers? Then I've listed it in both categories (like almonds: great source of calcium and protein!). Don't see a food you love on the following pages? No problem. I've crafted this list so that you can have a quick cheat sheet of the foods that are most rich in fat releasers. It's a resource—a place to eyeball the sorts of foods you should be reaching for with some regularity. It's a list you'll especially need after the 21-day plan is finished and you're committed to eating the Digest Diet way for life. If you're ever in doubt about whether a food fits the bill, this is the place to look.

Let's dig in.

Vitamin C

People who have inadequate levels of C cling more tightly to fat. Fruits and veggies can put you in release mode.

Top Choices

▶ Vegetables

Asparagus

Bell peppers, red and green

Broccoli

Broccoli rabe

Brussels sprouts

Cabbage

Cauliflower

Collard, mustard, and
    turnip greens

Escarole

Garlic

Kale

Kohlrabi

Onions

Peas, sugar snap

Spinach

Squash, summer and winter

Sweet potatoes

▶ Fruits

Cantaloupe

Grapefruit and fresh juice

Kiwifruit

Lemons

Limes

Mango

Oranges and fresh juice

Papaya

Pineapple

Raspberries

Strawberries

Tomatoes

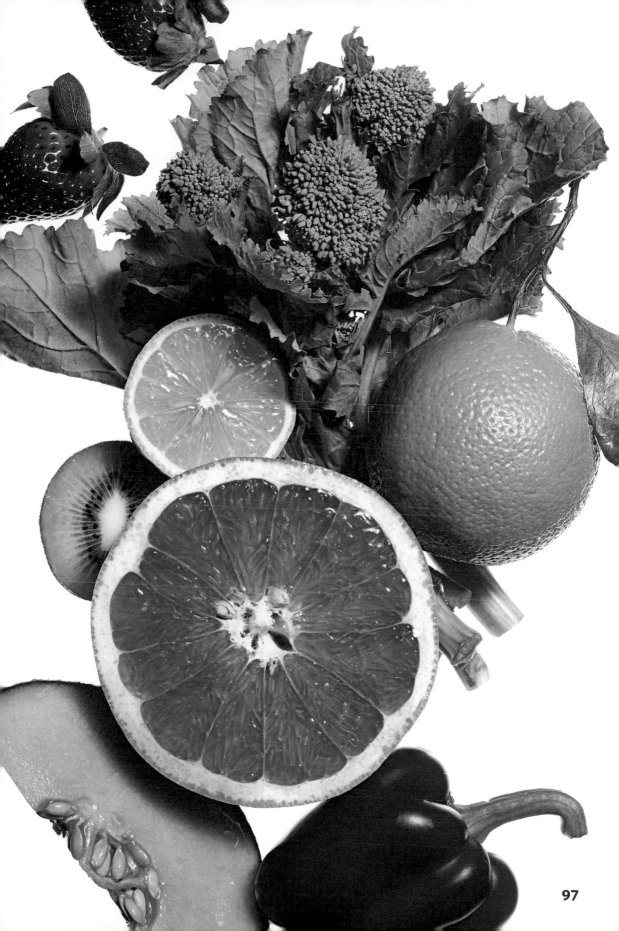

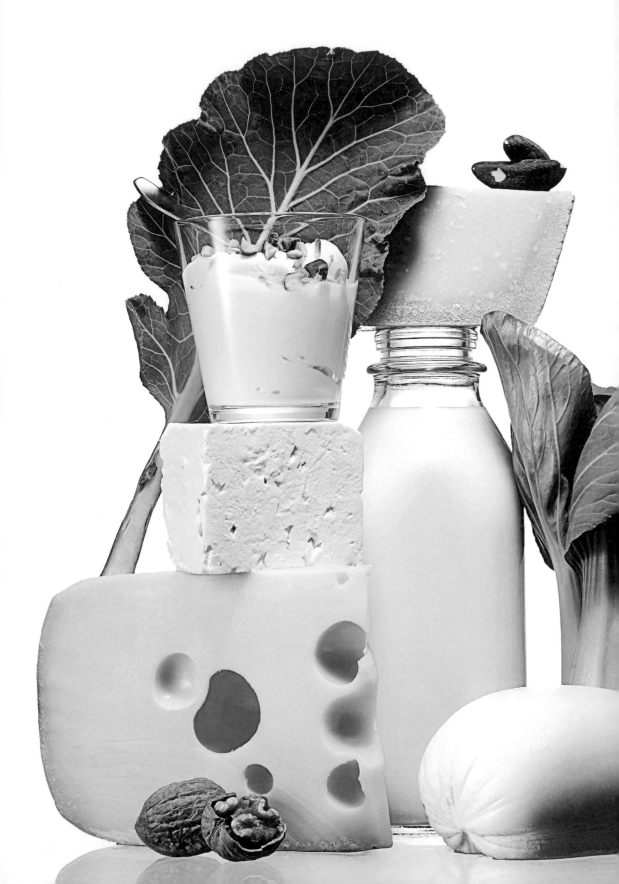

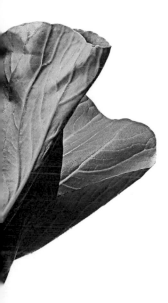

Calcium & Dairy

People deficient in calcium have a greater fat mass and increased hunger. Dairy foods are especially effective in accelerating fat loss.

Top Choices

▶ Dairy

Buttermilk

Cheddar cheese

Cottage cheese

Cream cheese

Feta cheese

Gruyère

Milk

Mozzarella cheese

Parmesan cheese

Provolone cheese

Ricotta cheese

Swiss cheese

Yogurt

▶ Nuts and Seeds

Almonds or almond
   butter

Brazil nuts

Roasted sesame
   seeds or sesame
   butter

▶ Vegetables

Bok choy

Broccoli

Broccoli rabe

Greens (collard,
   dandelion, turnip,
   and mustard)

Kale

Spinach

Watercress

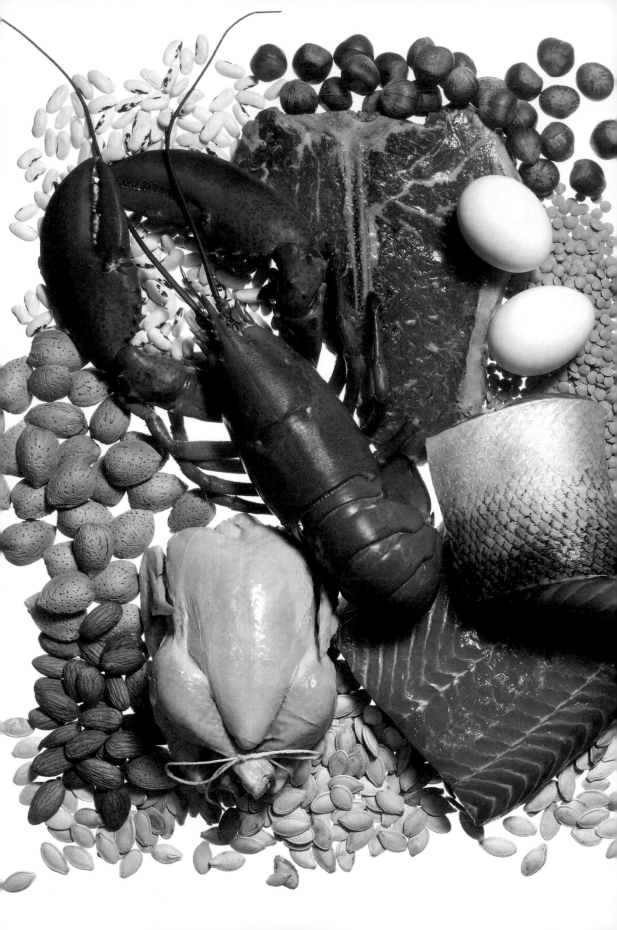

Protein

Protein increases feelings of satisfaction and fullness after a meal and boosts fat burn as well.

Top Choices

❯ Beans and Legumes

Baby lima beans

Lentils

Soybeans

White beans

❯ Dairy

See Dairy section
(page 99)

❯ Grains

Barley

Bread and tortillas,
whole-wheat

Couscous,
whole-wheat

Oats

❯ Nuts and Seeds

Almonds and
almond butter

Hazelnuts

Peanuts and peanut
butter

Pistachios

Pumpkin, squash,
or watermelon
seeds, roasted

❯ Poultry

Chicken

Eggs

Turkey

❯ Meats (lean cuts)

Beef

Pork

Veal

❯ Fish

Anchovies, fresh

Cod

Crab

Halibut

Lobster

Salmon, canned
and fresh

Sardines, canned
and fresh

Shrimp

Tuna, canned
and fresh

Healthy Fats

PUFAs may increase your resting metabolism, while MUFAs and coconut oil may help slim your belly faster.

Top Choices

Avocado

Coconut milk

Olive oil

Salmon

Sardines

Soybean oil

Sunflower oil

Nuts, seeds, and nut
butters, particularly
flax, walnut, and
sunflower

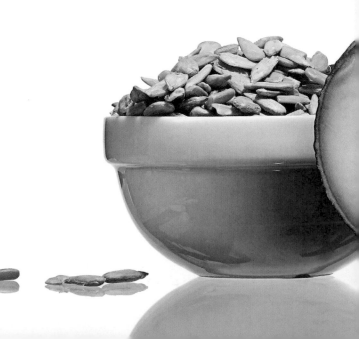

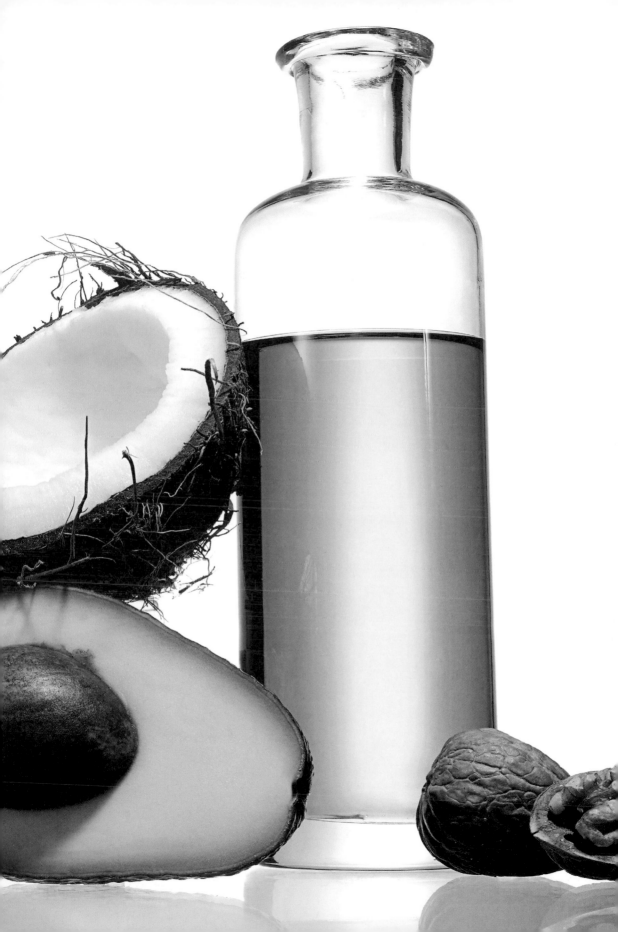

Quinoa

Animals that consume an extract from quinoa seeds decrease their body fat and food consumption. Plus, this grain is a good source of protein.

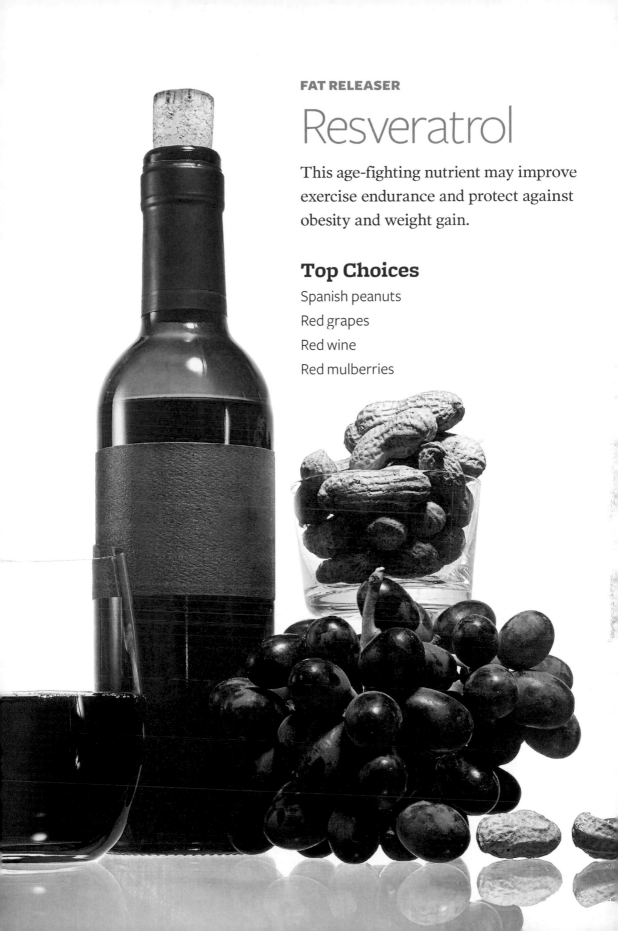

FAT RELEASER

Resveratrol

This age-fighting nutrient may improve exercise endurance and protect against obesity and weight gain.

Top Choices

Spanish peanuts

Red grapes

Red wine

Red mulberries

Cocoa

A small daily amount of cocoa or dark chocolate might blunt fat deposition—plus it strengthens our hearts, boosts mood, and keeps our skin young.

FAT RELEASER

Honey

In animal studies, honey has shown
great promise for reducing weight
gain and body fat.

Top Choices

Alfalfa

Avocado

Blueberry

Buckwheat

Clover

Manuka

Orange blossom

Tupelo

Wildflower

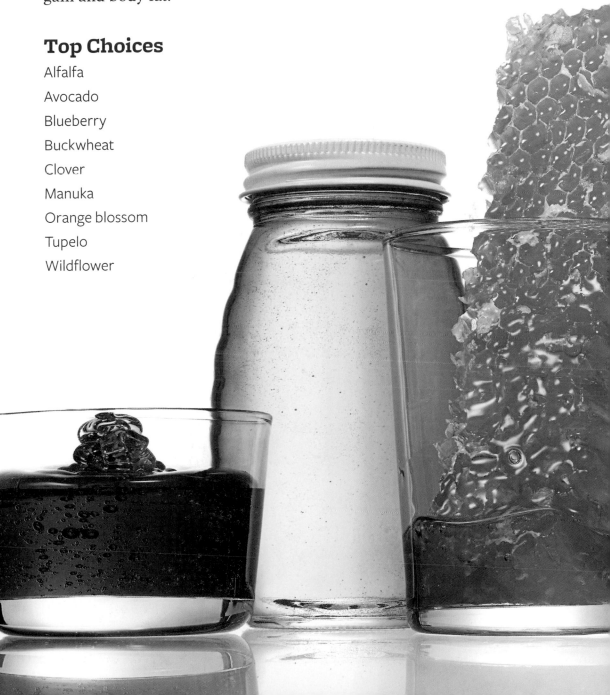

Fiber

Nothing fills you up—and prevents overeating—quite like fiber. It's found in so many whole foods, and it's easy to find delicious ways to add it to your meals.

Top Choices

▶ Fruits

Avocado

Blackberries

Plums

Raspberries

Tomatoes (fresh and
   sun-dried)

▶ Nuts and
   Seeds

Almonds

Brazil nuts

Flaxseed and
   flaxseed meal

Pistachios

Pecans

Sesame seeds

Sunflower seeds

▶ Grains

Barley

Couscous,
   whole-wheat

Rice, brown

Oats

▶ Legumes

Beans

Chickpeas

Edamame

Lentils

Peas, dried, fresh,
   snow, and sugar
   snap

▶ Vegetables

Artichokes

Broccoli rabe

Lettuce

Mustard greens

Radishes

Turnip greens

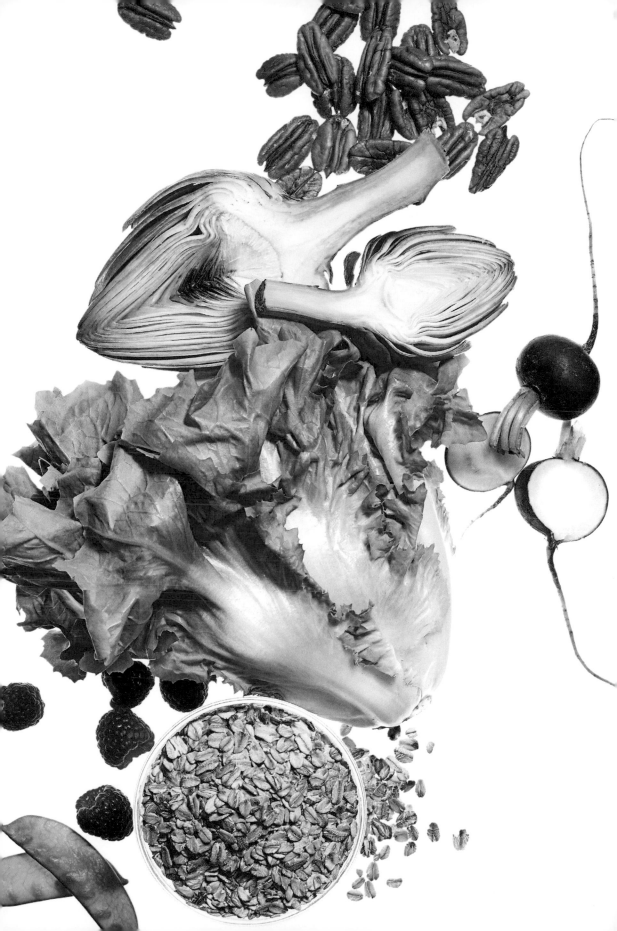

Vinegar

Mice that feed on a vinegar extract accumulate less body fat. Vinegar may also help prevent blood sugar spikes after meals.

Top Choices

Apple-cider

Balsamic

Malt

Red-wine

Rice

White, distilled

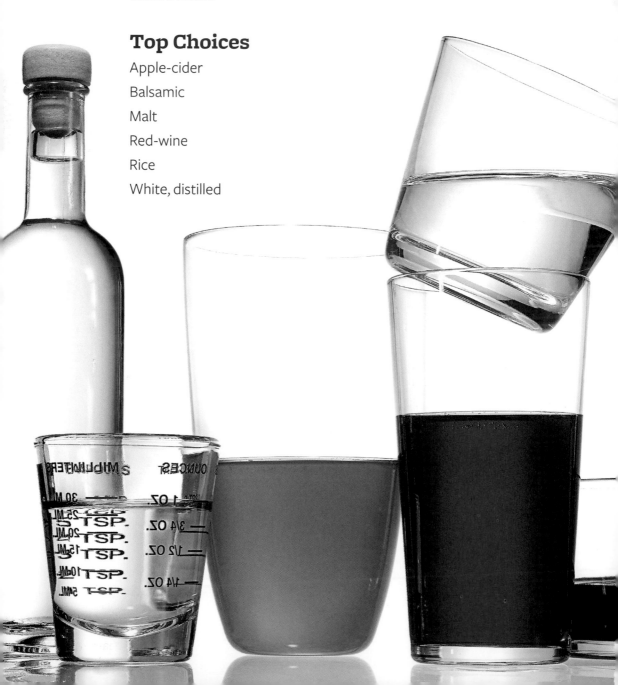

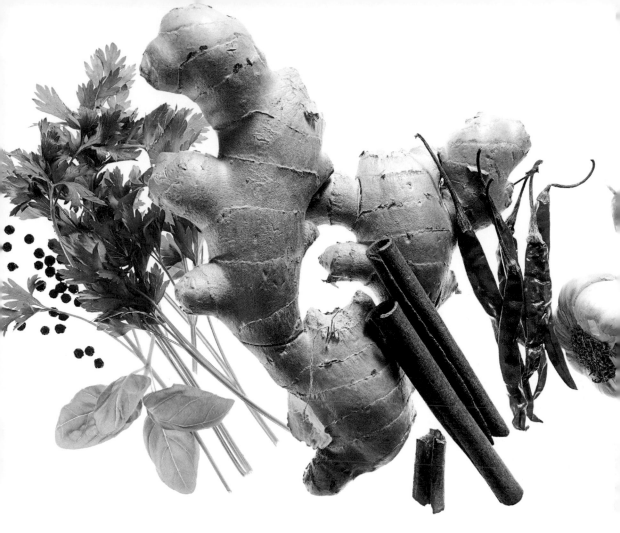

Fat Releaser Seasonings

These herbs and spices have modest amounts of multiple fat releasers. The exceptions are garlic and onions, as they are both terrific sources of C. The more you sprinkle these in, the better your food tastes, and the more fat releasers you consume.

Top Choices

Basil	Chile peppers	Marjoram	Red pepper flakes
Black pepper	Cinnamon	Onion	Rosemary
Cayenne pepper	Garlic	Oregano	Scallion
Celery seeds	Ginger	Parsley	Thyme

Chapter

5

"I am actually craving greens now!! That is ultra-exciting."

—ADRIENNE FARR,
LOST 18 POUNDS

Daily Fat Release Menus

Take advantage of the exciting science around fat releasing foods and behaviors. Slim down in three easy weeks!

N

ow that we know why and what we should be eating to release fat quickly, it's time to dig into the next 21 days of deliciously slimming foods. In this chapter, we've prepared a roadmap for you to follow so you know exactly what to eat at each meal and snack. If you find that some of the menus have foods that you don't like, feel free to repeat the shakes, snacks, and meals that are your favorites. Just be sure that any swapping you do is within a stage, not between stages, as we've calorie-controlled and apportioned the macronutrients in each stage slightly differently. Always remember, as with all parts of this diet, choose what suits you best: your tastes, needs, and likes.

● MAKE IT EASIER

While we were testing the diet, a few questions came up from our panelists that inspired me to further refine the plan. So before you get started, keep these things in mind.

Prep ahead. If planning out your meals each day is an issue or a challenge, then try this trick: Spend Sunday afternoon prepping for the week ahead. That means chopping vegetables, precooking meats, making soups ahead of time, and freezing portions. This way, everything is ready to go

SIMPLIFY IT: HOW TO MIX AND MATCH MEALS

While I encourage you to follow the plan as it's written for the next three weeks, our test panel had a suggestion they thought could be valuable, so I thought I'd share it here before you begin. Those who were single or were the only family members following the diet wanted to have the ability to shop less or repeat more of the same meals and menus. So for those who want to spend as little time in the kitchen or supermarket as possible, try this:

▶ **Repeat any day's menu** you like for two or three days of the plan.

▶ **Do the same with shakes:** Stick with one you like throughout the stage, rather than making the different varieties.

▶ **Repeat favorite meals** or snacks from different menus. If you have a favorite meal or snack, feel free to substitute them here for the ones that you don't like. But if you're just wary because they're new, give the original recipe or meal a try first!

You won't get as much variety from eating this way—and the calories aren't quite as strictly controlled—but your prep time decreases and your costs, too. **To keep you losing at a good rate, make sure you swap only within phases, not between them.** If you like Day 1 from Fast Release, then stick with it for the whole phase, but don't add in foods or snacks or meals from Fade Away.

when you need it. Invest in a great insulated lunchbox so you can take any food you need with you to work. Make premeasured bags of nuts and seeds to keep at your desk.

Refrigerate premade shakes. If you're bringing shakes with you, make sure to keep them in the fridge and have a

PSYCH-YOU-UP SHOPPING SUGGESTIONS!

Below are healthy picks for a few key items—mini-cheeses and wraps. These brands are my go-to choices for prepared foods. For complete shopping lists for the 21-Day plan, go to readersdigest.com/digestdiet.

WRAPS

These particular brands and flavors are good sources of fiber and protein (key fat releasers).

- Aladdin Low-Carb Wheat Wrap: 110 calories, 6g fiber, 10g protein
- Damascus Bakeries Roll-Up (flax): 110 calories, 9g fiber, 12g protein
- Damascus Bakeries Roll-Up (whole wheat): 110 calories, 7g fiber, 10g protein
- Flatout Flatbread (multigrain with flax): 100 calories, 8g fiber, 9g protein
- Flatout Flatbread (whole grain white): 110 calories, 7g fiber, 8g protein
- Flatout Flatbread Light (original): 90 calories, 9g fiber, 9g protein
- La Tortilla Factory Smart & Delicious Large Size Tortilla (whole wheat): 80 calories, 12g fiber, 8g protein

shaker cup to remix as needed. If you don't keep them cold, the testers found that they got lumpy and, as one tester said, thick enough to eat with a spoon.

Enjoy your daily caffeine. If you normally drink coffee, tea, or other caffeinated beverages and you stop doing so for

- La Tortilla Factory Smart & Delicious SoftWraps (multigrain): 100 calories, 12g fiber, 9g protein
- La Tortilla Factory Smart & Delicious Extra Virgin Olive Oil Soft Wraps (whole grain white): 100 calories, 13g fiber, 8g protein
- South Beach Diet (whole wheat): 110 calories, 8g fiber, 5g protein
- Tumaro's Gourmet Tortillas (multigrain): 100 calories, 8g fiber, 7g protein

MINI CHEESES

These reduced-fat cheeses come in tidy single-serving portions: convenient and calorie-controlled!

- The Laughing Cow Mini Babybel Light: 50 calories
- The Laughing Cow Light (any flavor): 35 calories
- Les Petites Fermieres Reduced-Fat Cheddar Cheese Sticks: 60 calories
- Sargento Reduced-Fat Colby-Jack Stick: 70 calories
- Polly-O 2% Mozzarella & Cheddar Cheese Twist: 50 calories

CRACKERS

Buy any brand that has about 30 calories and at least 1.5 grams of fiber per cracker. The ingredients list should contain "whole" ingredients, such as whole wheat, whole oats, etc.

the plan, you may develop a headache in the first few days. To avoid this rebound headache, feel free to drink one cup a day of your caffeinated beverage of choice, with one exception: No soda! And for a sweetener, use honey, as it's a fat releaser. If you don't like honey, then stick to no more than one teaspoon of raw or turbinado sugar. (Again: No artificial sweeteners.) What about cream in your coffee? It's best to use a splash of skim milk or, for a creamier texture, a skim-plus milk (great calcium source at 39 milligrams, too!). But no fake creamers or fat-free half-and-half—they make up for the fat by adding a lot of corn syrup.

Substitute your no-go foods. If you are allergic to a particular food or you just don't like it, swap it for a meal or snack within the same phase; you also have the option of repeating a day's menu.

If you have trouble tolerating dairy foods, substitute in coconut milk or almond or other nut milks. (However, we do encourage you to give dairy a fair try if you're not allergic or lactose intolerant. It is one of the most important and effective fat releasers.)

If you are allergic to a certain type of fish, then substitute 4 ounces of a lean chicken, turkey, beef, or pork or 6 ounces of a different lean fish that you can eat or do like (such as cod, sole, or tilapia).

If you don't like a snack or shake, go with your preferences and simply repeat what works for you within each phase. The same holds true for any other meals, snacks, or shakes.

If, say, you prefer red peppers to green, have at 'em. Just remember to keep the "thrive in five" tip (page 83) in mind, and check out the Fat Releaser Food Lists (pages 96–111) when choosing other nutrient-rich substitutes.

If you are a salt fan. Step away from the salt shaker and use a Fat Releaser Seasoning instead (see page 111). Another neat trick, when you're craving sodium: Squeeze the juice from a lemon or lime wedge over your meal.

If you are a soda fan. Much like trans fats, this is one area where there's nothing good in it for you. But if you just have to have something bubbly, have one glass of seltzer per day and generously squeeze in lemon or lime juice.

● DAILY ACTIVITY DIARY

On each day, I've written a reminder of what fat-burning moves (see Chapter 7) to work into your day. You'll also see a reminder—Don't forget to laugh!—because it's easy to use food as a substitute for fun. I also encourage you to take note of what other emotions send you straight to the fridge. When your kids frustrate you, do you reach for another helping? Or does a conversation with a parent have you worried, so you unconsciously grab for the candy and cookies? Only you can identify what is pulling you away from caring for yourself and embracing joy and fun. Go to readersdigest.com/digestdiet for a diary page that you can print to keep track of these moments. Whenever you can, write down how you're feeling and think of ways to address it. That puts the power where it belongs, in your hands . . . not in your food choices.

Let's get started!

THE 21-DAY PLAN

PHASE 1: DAYS 1–4
FAST RELEASE

Flood your body with nutrition:
Phase 1 fills you up on liquid shakes
and soups that are rich in vitamins,
minerals, and protein, to gently coax
your body into quick, safe weight loss.
(Our top tester lost 10 pounds during
this phase!)

Eating Rules

▶ Drink 2 Fast Release Shakes a day (see
recipe on page 153). One at breakfast,
to start the day off right; the second,
you can choose to have as your lunch
or dinner meal.

▶ Snack once a day.

▶ Have a 2-cup serving of soup for
lunch or dinner. See pages 163–171
for a variety of soup recipes.

▶ Space meals according to your needs,
but try to go no longer than four
hours between eating.

PHASE 2: DAYS 5–14
FADE AWAY

Go lean and green: That's the theme
of this 10-day phase in which you'll
continue to enjoy steady weight loss,
while enjoying a Mediterranean-style
diet rich in lean protein, healthy fats,
and a bounty of vegetables. And yes:
You get to enjoy a glass of red wine
with dinner, if you like.

Eating Rules

▶ Drink first, eat second.

▶ Have 1 Fade Away Shake a day (see
recipe on page 155).

▶ Think lean and green when making
choices.

▶ Eat healthy fats (MUFAs and PUFAs).

▶ Snack twice a day.

▶ Enjoy a glass of wine or a handful of
red grapes at dinner.

PHASE 3: DAYS 15–21
FINISH STRONG

Eat a balanced diet for life: That's what Phase 3 teaches you as you enjoy a wider variety of foods (such as pizza, pasta, and bread), while consuming proper portions of carbs, proteins, and healthy fats. And, of course, every meal will contain a number of healthy fat releasing foods! This phase helps you both reach your goal weight and maintain what you've lost.

Eating Rules

▶ Continue to drink first, eat second.

▶ Continue to snack twice a day.

▶ Continue to enjoy a glass of red wine with dinner.

▶ Enjoy a dessert or favorite treat once a week.

▶ Bring a balanced eye.

MAKE GROCERY SHOPPING A SNAP!!

To get a grocery list for all three phases of the plan, go to readersdigest.com/digestdiet. You'll be able to customize it with the foods and meals you like, plus keep track of favorites for easier shopping.

HELPFUL HINT
FOLLOW OUR SERVING SIZES

Pay careful attention to serving sizes as you read through the plan. The 21-Day Plan gives individual portions. However, the recipes serve 4 (and in the case of soups, up to 8). This is so those of you cooking for families or who wish to make and freeze meals ahead can do so. To be sure you are eating single servings, follow the portion guide at the bottom of the recipes (where the nutritional information is given).

DAY 1 FAST RELEASE

Breakfast

Fast Release Shake (page 153)

Snack

Ricotta Boats: Cut a green bell pepper into quarters and seed. Top each with 2 tablespoons fat-free ricotta cheese and a couple of good grinds of black pepper.

Lunch

Fast Release Shake (page 153) or 2-cup serving of **Soup** (choose from pages 163–171)

Dinner

Fast Release Shake (page 153) or 2-cup serving of **Soup** (choose from pages 163–171)

ACTIVITY PLANNER

☐ **Morning Moves.** Take a 45- to 60-minute walk. We won't begin the Fat Release Workout until Day 5. Feel free to break up the walk into smaller increments, as needed or desired, throughout the plan.

☐ **1-Minute Activity Bursts.** Do three. Choose from the activities on pages 256–257 or do whatever moves you.

☐ **Don't forget to laugh!**

DAY 2 FAST RELEASE

Breakfast
Fast Release Shake (page 153)

Snack
Cheesy Rollup: 1 reduced-fat mozzarella stick rolled up in 2 large, crunchy romaine lettuce leaves

Lunch
Fast Release Shake (page 153) or 2-cup serving of **Soup** (choose from pages 163–171)

Dinner
Fast Release Shake (page 153) or 2-cup serving of **Soup** (choose from pages 163–171)

ACTIVITY PLANNER

☐ **Morning Moves.** Take a 45- to 60-minute walk. Feel free to break up the walk into smaller increments, as needed or desired, throughout the plan.

☐ **1-Minute Activity Bursts.** Do three. Choose from the activities on pages 256–257 or do whatever moves you.

☐ **Don't forget to laugh!**

DAY 3 FAST RELEASE

Breakfast
Fast Release Shake (page 153)

Snack
Tomato Cream Spread: Stir 4 finely chopped grape tomatoes into ¼ cup fat-free cream cheese. Season with a pinch of oregano and black pepper to taste. Spread on pieces of celery or fresh fennel.

Lunch
Fast Release Shake (page 153) or 2-cup serving of **Soup** (choose from pages 163–171)

Dinner
Fast Release Shake (page 153) or 2-cup serving of **Soup** (choose from pages 163–171)

ACTIVITY PLANNER

☐ **Morning Moves.** Take a 45- to 60-minute walk. Feel free to break up the walk into smaller increments, as needed or desired, throughout the plan.

☐ **1-Minute Activity Bursts.** Do three. Choose from the activities on pages 256–257 or do whatever moves you.

☐ **Don't forget to laugh!**

DAY 4 FAST RELEASE

Breakfast

Fast Release Shake (page 153)

Snack

Tangy Yogurt Dip: Stir together ½ cup 0% Greek yogurt and ½ teaspoon olive oil. Season with a pinch of curry powder or chili powder, and black pepper to taste. Serve with raw or lightly steamed broccoli or cauliflower florets or green beans for dipping.

Lunch

Fast Release Shake (page 153) or 2-cup serving of **Soup** (choose from pages 163–171)

Dinner

Fast Release Shake (page 153) or 2-cup serving of **Soup** (choose from pages 163–171)

ACTIVITY PLANNER

☐ **Morning Moves.** Take a 45- to 60-minute walk. Feel free to break up the walk into smaller increments, as needed or desire, throughout the plan.

☐ **1-Minute Activity Bursts.** Do three. Choose from the activities on pages 256–257 or do whatever moves you.

☐ **Don't forget to laugh!**

DAY 5   FADE AWAY

Breakfast
Creamy Quinoa (page 159)

Snack
Mixed Munchies: ½ cup nonfat yogurt (with a Fat Releaser Seasoning, page 111, if desired), 1 tablespoon sunflower seeds, and 10 baby carrots

Lunch
Fade Away Shake (page 155)

Snack
Mixed Munchies: 20 pistachios and 10 baby carrots; serve with ½ cup fat-free milk.

Dinner
Pork and Pepper Plate: 4-ounce broiled boneless pork chop and Peperonata with Fennel (page 219). Have a 4-ounce glass of red wine with dinner or a handful of red grapes for dessert.

ACTIVITY PLANNER

☐ **Morning Moves.** Perform the 12-Minute Fat Release Workout from page 246 and take a 20-minute walk.

☐ **1-Minute Activity Bursts.** Do three (pages 256–257).

☐ **Don't forget to laugh!**

DAY 6 FADE AWAY

Breakfast
Fade Away Shake (page 155)

Snack
Mixed Munchies: 1 mini cheese (see page 117), 20 pistachios, and 3 celery stalks

Lunch
Turkey & Cheddar Rollup: Combine 1 tablespoon 0% Greek yogurt with 1 teaspoon Dijon mustard and spread it on a high-fiber wrap (see pages 116–117). Add 1 cup baby spinach leaves, arugula, or field greens, 2 ounces sliced lower-sodium deli roast turkey, and 1 ounce reduced-fat cheddar cheese. Roll it up and eat as is, or warm it in the toaster oven or microwave. Enjoy with ½ cup fat-free milk.

Snack
PB & Crackers: 2 teaspoons natural peanut butter and 2 whole-grain crackers (see page 117); serve with ½ cup fat-free milk.

Dinner
Shrimp Plate: 6 ounces grilled shrimp, Edamame Mash with Parmesan (page 218), and 2 cups baby spinach tossed with 1 tablespoon Digest Diet Vinaigrette (page 211). Have a 4-ounce glass of red wine with dinner or a handful of red grapes for dessert.

ACTIVITY PLANNER

❑ **Morning Moves.** Walk for 45 to 60 minutes.

❑ **1-Minute Activity Bursts.** Do three (pages 256–257).

❑ **Don't forget to laugh!**

DAY 7 FADE AWAY

Breakfast

Mexilicious Omelet (page 158) and 1 cup fat-free milk

Snack

PB & Carrots: 1 tablespoon natural peanut butter and 10 baby carrots

Lunch

Fade Away Shake (page 155)

Snack

Mixed Munchies: 1 mini cheese, 20 pistachios, and ½ cup grape tomatoes

Dinner

Big-Batch Roast Chicken (pages 173–174), 2 cups steamed broccoli, and 2 cups field greens tossed with 1 tablespoon Digest Diet Vinaigrette (page 211). Have a 4-ounce glass of red wine with dinner or a handful of red grapes for dessert.

ACTIVITY PLANNER

☐ **Morning Moves.** Rest. Take this time to go have some fun!

☐ **Don't forget to laugh!**

DAY 8 FADE AWAY

Breakfast
Fade Away Shake (page 155)

Snack
Mixed Munchies: 1 mini cheese, ½ cup grape tomatoes, and 10 almonds

Lunch
Chicken-Cabbage Salad: Blend 2 teaspoons natural peanut butter, 2 teaspoons vinegar, 1 tablespoon water, a small pinch each of sea salt and cayenne pepper. Toss with 4 ounces shredded, cooked chicken breast and 2 cups coleslaw mix. Enjoy with 1 cup fat-free milk.

Snack
Nutty Yogurt Spread: Combine ½ cup nonfat yogurt (with a Fat Releaser Seasoning, page 111, if desired) with 1 tablespoon sunflower seeds and spread on bell pepper slices (1 pepper).

Dinner
Tri-Color Frittata (page 197), plus 2 cups shredded romaine tossed with 1 tablespoon Digest Diet Vinaigrette (page 211) and 2 teaspoons shredded Parmesan cheese. Have a 4-ounce glass of red wine with dinner or a handful of red grapes for dessert.

ACTIVITY PLANNER

☐ **Morning Moves.** Perform the 12-Minute Fat Release Workout from page 246 and take a 20-minute walk.

☐ **1-Minute Activity Bursts.** Do three (pages 256–257).

☐ **Don't forget to laugh!**

Breakfast

Scrambled Egg & Bacon Wrap: Whisk together 1 whole egg and 1 egg white (or 6 tablespoons egg substitute) and scramble with 1 small chopped slice of Canadian bacon in a pan sprayed lightly with olive oil. Roll up in a high-fiber wrap spread with 2 tablespoons fat-free cream cheese and sprinkled with a Fat Releaser Seasoning (page 111). Enjoy with 1 cup fat-free milk.

Snack

Ricotta Dip: Combine ¼ cup fat-free ricotta cheese (with a Fat Releaser Seasoning, page 111, if desired) with 1 tablespoon sunflower seeds. Enjoy as a dip with 10 baby carrots.

Lunch

Fade Away Shake (page 155)

Snack

Mixed Munchies: 1 mini cheese, 20 pistachios, and 2 celery stalks

Dinner

Steak Out!: 3 ounces grilled flank steak, 2 cups grilled summer squash, Orange-Chipotle Broccoli Rabe (page 225). Have a 4-ounce glass of red wine with dinner or a handful of red grapes for dessert.

ACTIVITY PLANNER

☐ **Morning Moves.** Walk for 45 to 60 minutes.

☐ **1-Minute Activity Bursts.** Do three (pages 256–257).

☐ **Don't forget to laugh!**

Breakfast

Fade Away Shake (page 155)

Snack

Mixed Munchies: ½ cup nonfat yogurt (with a Fat Releaser Seasoning, page 111, if desired), ½ red bell pepper (seeded and sliced), 20 pistachios

Lunch

Soup: One-cup serving of leftovers you froze, or make a new one (pages 163–171). Enjoy with 2 whole-grain crackers, 1 ounce reduced-fat cheddar cheese, and 1 cup fat-free milk.

Snack

Ricotta Dip: Combine ¼ cup fat-free ricotta cheese (with a Fat Releaser Seasoning, page 111, if desired) with 2 teaspoons sunflower seeds. Enjoy as a dip with 10 baby carrots.

Dinner

Turkey-Mushroom Burger (page 180) and Japanese Spinach Sal ad with Carrot-Sesame Dressing (page 201). Have a 4-ounce glass of red wine with dinner or a handful of red grapes for dessert.

ACTIVITY PLANNER

☐ **Morning Moves.** Perform the 12-Minute Fat Release Workout from page 246 and take a 20-minute walk.

☐ **1-Minute Activity Bursts.** Do three (pages 256–257).

☐ **Don't forget to laugh!**

Breakfast

Creamy Quinoa (page 159)

Snack

PB & Crackers: 2 teaspoons natural peanut butter and 2 whole-grain crackers; serve with ½ cup fat-free milk.

Lunch

Fade Away Shake (page 155)

Snack

Yogurt Dip: ½ red bell pepper (seeded and sliced), ½ cup nonfat yogurt (with a Fat Releaser Seasoning, page 111, if desired), and 10 almonds

Dinner

Balsamic Glazed Salmon (page 193), 2 cups steamed asparagus, and 2 cups field greens tossed with 1 tablespoon Digest Diet Vinaigrette (page 211). Have a 4-ounce glass of red wine with dinner or a handful of red grapes for dessert.

ACTIVITY PLANNER

☐ **Morning Moves.** Walk for 45 to 60 minutes.

☐ **1-Minute Activity Bursts.** Do three (pages 256–257).

☐ **Don't forget to laugh!**

FADE AWAY

Breakfast

Fade Away Shake (page 155)

Snack

Mixed Munchies: 1 mini cheese, 10 baby carrots, and 8 almonds

Lunch

Tuna, Egg & Chickpea Salad with Buttermilk Dressing
(page 203)

Snack

PB & Crackers: 2 teaspoons natural peanut butter and
2 whole-grain crackers; serve with ½ cup fat-free milk.

Dinner

Braised Chicken with Artichokes and Sun-Dried Tomatoes
(page 177) and 2 cups field greens tossed with 1 tablespoon Digest
Diet Vinaigrette (page 211). Have a 4-ounce glass of red wine with
dinner or a handful of red grapes for dessert.

ACTIVITY PLANNER

☐ **Morning Moves.** Perform the 12-Minute Fat Release Workout
from page 246 and take a 20-minute walk.

☐ **1-Minute Activity Bursts.** Do three (pages 256–257).

☐ **Don't forget to laugh!**

Breakfast

Egg Cup: Cut the top inch off a green bell pepper; remove ribs and seeds. Stuff with a small handful of baby spinach or arugula, 1 ounce reduced-sodium deli roast turkey or ham, and 2 tablespoons shredded reduced-fat cheese. Top with an egg and a pinch of black pepper. Pierce the yolk and replace the pepper top. Microwave for 4 to 5 minutes. Let sit, covered, for 3 minutes. Enjoy with 1 cup fat-free milk.

Snack

Mixed Munchies: ½ cup grape tomatoes, ¼ cup fat-free ricotta cheese, and 1 tablespoon sunflower seeds

Lunch

Fade Away Shake (page 155)

Snack

Mixed Munchies: 1 mini cheese, 20 pistachios, and 2 celery stalks

Dinner

Festive Fish: 6 ounces broiled cod, 2 cups steamed green beans, and Watercress-Arugula Salad with Parmesan "Crackers" (page 209). Have a 4-ounce glass of red wine with dinner or a handful of red grapes for dessert.

ACTIVITY PLANNER

☐ **Morning Moves.** Walk for 45 to 60 minutes.

☐ **1-Minute Activity Bursts.** Do three (pages 256–257).

☐ **Don't forget to laugh!**

Breakfast
Fade Away Shake (page 155)

Snack
Mixed Munchies: 1 mini cheese, 10 almonds, and ½ red bell pepper

Lunch
Turkey-Asparagus Rollups: Spread 4 ounces reduced-sodium deli turkey with 2 teaspoons Dijon mustard and wrap around 6 cooked asparagus spears. Serve with 1 sliced tomato and 1 cup fat-free milk.

Snack
Mixed Munchies: ½ cup nonfat yogurt (with a Fat Releaser Seasoning, page 111), 1 tablespoon pumpkin seeds, and 10 baby carrots

Dinner
Portabella Panini: Scrape the gills out of 2 portabella mushrooms; brush with balsamic vinegar. Cook, gill-side down, in an electric grill or sandwich press until softened. Flip and top with 1 ounce Jarlsberg light cheese and 2 ounces (about 2 slices) reduced-sodium deli ham. Top with the second mushroom and cook until the cheese melts. Serve with 1½ cups coleslaw mix tossed with 2 tablespoons nonfat yogurt and 1 tablespoon Digest Diet Vinaigrette (page 211). Have a 4-ounce glass of red wine with dinner or a handful of red grapes for dessert.

ACTIVITY PLANNER

☐ **Morning Moves.** Rest. Take this time to go have some fun!

☐ **Don't forget to laugh!**

Breakfast

California Dream Omelet (page 158), ½ cup fat-free milk, and 2 slices (½-inch) toasted whole-grain baguette

Snack

Mixed Munchies: ¼ cup fat-free ricotta cheese (with a Fat Releaser Seasoning, page 111, if desired), 5 grape tomatoes, and 5 almonds

Lunch

Soup: 1-cup serving of a leftover soup, or make a new one (pages 163–171), 2 whole-grain crackers, and 1 cup fat-free milk

Snack

PB & D: 2 teaspoons natural peanut butter and 2 dates

Dinner

Big-Batch Roast Chicken (pages 173–174), 2 cups steamed broccoli, ½ cup whole-wheat couscous (page 227), and 2 cups shredded romaine lettuce tossed with 1 tablespoon Digest Diet Vinaigrette (page 211). Have a 4-ounce glass of red wine with dinner or a handful of red grapes for dessert.

ACTIVITY PLANNER

☐ **Morning Moves.** Perform the 12-Minute Fat Release Workout (reverse order) from page 246 and take a 20-minute walk.

☐ **1-Minute Activity Bursts.** Do three to five (pages 256–257).

☐ **Don't forget to laugh!**

Breakfast

1 Oatmeal Breakfast Cake (page 157), ½ cup nonfat yogurt, and 1 orange

Snack

PB & Crackers: 2 teaspoons natural peanut butter, 2 whole-grain crackers, and 2 tablespoons unsweetened applesauce

Lunch

Spicy Blender Gazpacho: Coarsely chop together 2 plum tomatoes, ½ cucumber, ⅛ small red onion, 2 tablespoons flaxseed meal, cayenne pepper (to taste), and red-wine vinegar (to taste). Serve with 4 slices (½-inch) toasted whole-wheat baguette and ½ cup fat-free milk.

Snack

Mixed Munchies: 1 mini cheese and 1 apple

Dinner

Chunky Beef & Vegetable Chili with Red Wine (page 189), ½ cup cooked brown rice (pages 228–229), and 2 cups field greens tossed with 1 tablespoon Digest Diet Vinaigrette (page 211).

ACTIVITY PLANNER

☐ **Morning Moves.** Walk for 60 minutes.

☐ **1-Minute Activity Bursts.** Do three to five (pages 256–257).

☐ **Don't forget to laugh!**

Breakfast

Peanut Butter and Almost Jelly Rollup: Spread a high-fiber wrap with 1 tablespoon natural peanut butter. Top with chopped fruit: 1 kiwi, ½ cup strawberries, or ½ cup red grapes. Roll up and enjoy.

Snack

Ricotta Cup: Stir 2 chopped dates into ¼ cup fat-free ricotta cheese and add cinnamon to taste.

Lunch

Chicken & Broccoli Salad: Toss 3 ounces shredded cooked chicken breast with 2 cups chopped cooked broccoli, 1 tablespoon chopped toasted walnuts, 1 tablespoon Digest Diet Vinaigrette (page 211), 2 tablespoons nonfat yogurt, and 1 tablespoon water. Serve with 2 slices (½-inch) whole-wheat baguette.

Snack

Creamy Fruit Cup: 1 chopped nectarine tossed with ¼ cup nonfat yogurt and 1 teaspoon honey

Dinner

Pizza with Wilted Greens, Ricotta & Almonds (page 199) and 2 cups field greens tossed with 1 tablespoon Digest Diet Vinaigrette (page 211). Have 4 ounces of red wine or a handful of red grapes.

ACTIVITY PLANNER

☐ **Morning Moves.** Perform the 12-Minute Fat Release Workout (reverse order) from page 246 and take a 20-minute walk.

☐ **1-Minute Activity Bursts.** Do three to five (pages 256–257).

☐ **Don't forget to laugh!**

DAY 18 FINISH STRONG

Breakfast

Oatmeal: ½ cup quick-cooking oats cooked according to package directions with 1 cup unsweetened almond milk. Top with 4 sliced strawberries, 1 tablespoon sliced almonds, and 2 teaspoons honey.

Snack

Creamy Fruit Cup: 1 chopped pear tossed with ¼ cup nonfat yogurt and 1 teaspoon honey

Lunch

Couscous Salad: Toss together ½ cup cooked whole-wheat couscous (page 233), ¼ sliced avocado, ½ cup chopped oranges, 2 chopped scallions, 3 tablespoons reduced-fat goat cheese or feta cheese, and 2 teaspoons Digest Diet Vinaigrette (page 211).

Snack

Cheese & Crackers: 1 mini cheese, 1 kiwi, 2 whole-grain crackers

Dinner

Burger night!: Broiled turkey burger made with 3 ounces ground turkey breast and 1 ounce mashed chickpeas. Add a beefsteak tomato slice and make an open-face sandwich on 1 slice whole-grain peasant bread. Serve with Tangy Broccoli Slaw (page 207). Have 4 ounces of red wine or a handful of red grapes.

ACTIVITY PLANNER

☐ **Morning Moves.** Walk for 60 minutes.

☐ **1-Minute Activity Bursts.** Do three to five (pages 256–257).

☐ **Don't forget to laugh!**

Breakfast

California Dream Omelet (page 158), 2 slices (½-inch) toasted whole-wheat baguette, and ½ cup fat-free milk

Snack

Fast Fruit Cup: ½ cup blueberries topped with ¼ cup fat-free ricotta cheese and 5 almonds (chopped)

Lunch

Soup: 1-cup serving of a leftover soup, or make a new one (pages 163–171), 2 slices (1 ounce) toasted whole-wheat bread, and 1 cup fat-free milk

Snack

PB & O: 2 teaspoons natural peanut butter and 1 orange

Dinner

Spaghetti with Super Mushroomy Marinara (page 191). Have a 4-ounce glass of red wine with dinner or a handful of red grapes for dessert.

ACTIVITY PLANNER

☐ **Morning Moves.** Perform the 12-Minute Fat Release Workout (reverse order) from page 246 and take a 20-minute walk.

☐ **1-Minute Activity Bursts.** Do three to five (pages 256–257).

☐ **Don't forget to laugh!**

Breakfast

Honey-Nut Yogurt Parfait (page 161)

Snack

PB & A: 2 teaspoons natural peanut butter and 1 apple

Lunch

Kale Salad with Feta, Grapes & Pumpkin Seeds (page 204), 2 slices (½-inch) whole-wheat baguette, and 1 cup fat-free milk

Snack

Cheese & Crackers: 1 mini cheese and 2 whole-grain crackers

Dinner

Steak Plate: 3 ounces broiled flank steak, 2 cups steamed Chinese stir-fry vegetables, and Baked Sweet Potatoes with Peanut Sauce (page 224). Have a 4-ounce glass of red wine with dinner or a handful of red grapes for dessert.

ACTIVITY PLANNER

☐ **Morning Moves.** Walk for 60 minutes.

☐ **1-Minute Activity Bursts.** Do three to five (pages 256–257).

☐ **Don't forget to laugh!**

Breakfast

1 Oatmeal Breakfast Cake (page 157) topped with 2 tablespoons fat-free cream cheese and 2 tablespoons unsweetened applesauce and cinnamon to taste; serve with ½ cup fat-free milk.

Snack

Quick Yogurt Cup: Combine ½ cup nonfat yogurt, 1 tablespoon sunflower seeds, and 2 chopped dates.

Lunch

Spicy Blender Gazpacho: Coarsely chop together 2 plum tomatoes, ½ cucumber, ⅛ small red onion, 2 tablespoons flaxseed meal, cayenne pepper (to taste), and red-wine vinegar (to taste). Serve with 4 whole-grain crackers.

Snack

Mixed Munchies: 1 cup fat-free milk and ½ cup blueberries

Dinner

Baja Fish Tacos with Avocado-Radish Relish and "Crema" (page 192) and 1 Fudgy Mocha Brownie (page 237). Have a 4-ounce glass of red wine with dinner or a handful of red grapes for dessert.

ACTIVITY PLANNER

☐ **Morning Moves.** Rest. Take this time to have some fun!

☐ **Don't forget to laugh!**

Checking In

Want motivation to stick to the 21-Day Plan? I can't stress enough how helpful keeping a daily journal is. Here's a sample page to help you get started. Use it to track your successes, write down your feelings, and jot down ideas for how to overcome your challenges. Go to **readersdigest.com/digestdiet** to get a printable version to use every day.

What Made You Laugh Today?

_____

_____

_____

When, Where, and How Did You Move?

_____

_____

_____

What Challenged You?

_____

_____

_____

Balancing Act—What Can/Did You Do to Achieve More of It?

_____

_____

_____

Chapter

6

"My mom and I enjoyed making the recipes together, putting love into the food."

—DANA MIELE,
LOST 8 POUNDS

Fat Release Recipes

Dig into these 50 delicious dishes bursting with the foods that release fat. The whole family will love them!

I **have come to believe that cooking**—for yourself and for your family—is an act of love. You're caring for yourself. You're nourishing your children. You're selecting tastes and textures that you know your spouse will enjoy. You're preparing the centerpiece for one of the most important moments of the day—the time when (if even for a few minutes) everyone in your home sits down together. The family table. The family meal. Both are key to a happy, healthy home . . . to a happy, healthy you.

Even the act of washing a pint of raspberries on a Saturday morning, then putting them on a paper towel to dry, is an act of love. It feels great to watch my girls run in and out of the kitchen, picking up a little burst of nourishment as they pass.

The Digest Diet recipes have been created and tested with this specific double whammy in mind: They should give you both a burst of nourishment and a burst of flavor. I hope you'll find something tasty in each of the recipe sections, which I've organized like this:

1. Slimming Shakes
2. Breakfasts
3. Soups
4. Main Courses
5. Salads
6. Side Dishes
7. Desserts

Enjoy delicious breakfast ideas like the Creamy Quinoa or Mexilicious Omelet. Or warm yourself on a wintry day with Spiced Winter Squash Soup with Asian Greens. Cooking for dinner? Make up a Big-Batch Roast Chicken and be set for the week, or try the Chile-Rubbed Pork Tenderloin, Baked Sweet Potatoes with Peanut Sauce, and the Stir-Fried Asparagus and Scallions and wow your family and friends. My favorite dessert? Hard to pick: maybe the Banana Bonbons and the Milk Chocolate Cheesecakelets, but I am a huge fan of the Fudgy Mocha Brownies, too.

Whichever dishes turn out to be your favorites, they are meant to be enjoyed with family and friends, knowing the whole time that each bite is nourishing your body and tantalizing your taste buds.

● HOW TO GET THE MOST OUT OF THE FAT RELEASE RECIPES

Because I know firsthand just how busy life is, both the Fat Release Menus from Chapter 5 and all of the Fat Release Recipes within this chapter are simple to prepare and not terribly time-consuming.

Just as the menus walk you through simple ways to eat more fat releasers during the three weeks of the eating plan, each of the recipes in this chapter is chock-full of wholesome fat releasing foods. You can eyeball a dish and find out immediately which of your favorite fat releasers it has, as we've listed them right there for you. Also, each recipe gives you a breakdown of key macro- and micronutrients and fiber, as well as calories per serving.

The bulk of the recipes serve four people, with bigger

batches for the soups and some of the desserts. If you're single or your household is smaller than four, you can scale down the recipe or prepare it as called for and freeze and store for later use. Cook once; eat multiple times. Works for me! Say you want or need an even bigger batch? Scale it up (just keep to eating the same portion sizes—those don't change). I want these new dishes to become the standards in your household, to become the meals that you and your family enjoy around the table each day.

● AFTER THE 21-DAY DIET: CREATE YOUR OWN MENUS

After you finish the 21-Day Daily Fat Release Menus in Chapter 5, you'll probably want to branch out and add variety while continuing to lose (or maintaining your loss). I've included extra recipes in this chapter so you can have on hand new ideas for making the Digest Diet a way of life. At the bottom of each recipe, I've provided all the nutrition information you need to create a calorie-controlled menu that's loaded with key fat releasing nutrients. But if you need more guidance, start right here, with the three general principles you can follow to create Digest Diet meals.

1. Match a plain lean protein with a side-dish vegetable recipe

If you're modeling your menu after the Fade Away phase (Days 5 to 14), that means pairing 4 ounces of broiled, grilled, or roasted lean protein (chicken, beef, pork) or 6 ounces of broiled, grilled, or poached lean fish or shrimp with any of these dishes:

- ▶ **Stir-Fried Asparagus & Scallions** (page 213)
- ▶ **Spicy Braised Collards with Garlic & Raisins** (page 215)
- ▶ **Almond-Parmesan Cauliflower au Gratin** (page 217)
- ▶ **Olive Oil–Roasted Brussels Sprouts** (page 214)
- ▶ **Tangy Broccoli Slaw** (page 207)
- ▶ **Japanese Spinach Salad with Carrot-Sesame Dressing** (page 201)

If you're modeling your menu after the Finish Strong phase (Days 15 to 21) or are eating to maintain your loss, include these starchier side options:

- ▶ **Green Peas & Sautéed Shallots with Thai Herbs** (page 216)
- ▶ **Potatoes with Spicy Paprika-Pepper Sauce** (page 221)
- ▶ **Any of the couscous options** (page 227)
- ▶ **Any of the brown rice options** (pages 228–229)

2. Match a main-dish recipe with a plain vegetable side

If you're modeling your menu after the Fade Away phase (Days 5 to 14), you can match 2 cups steamed (or microwaved) nonstarchy vegetables (broccoli, cauliflower, green beans, peppers, eggplant, fennel, jicama, kale, spinach, collards, etc.) with any of these:

- ▶ **Marinated Flank Steak with Grilled Red Onions** (page 187)
- ▶ **Grilled Turkey Cutlets with Lemon & Marjoram** (page 183)
- ▶ **Chile-Rubbed Pork Tenderloin** (page 181)
- ▶ **Balsamic-Glazed Salmon** (page 193)
- ▶ **Poached Chicken with Garlic-Walnut Sauce** (page 175)
- ▶ **Citrus- & Herb-Marinated Pork Chops** (page 179)

If you're modeling your menu after the Finish Strong phase (Days 15 to 21) or are eating to maintain your loss, add a ½-cup serving of couscous or brown rice or 2 ounces of whole-grain bread.

3. Have a one-dish main

The following dishes have a healthy balance of protein, fat, and carbs to fit well into the Fade Away phase (Days 5 to 14); adding 2 cups of salad greens tossed with 1 tablespoon Digest Diet Vinaigrette (page 211) is a nutritious, low-cal, and filling way to round out your meal. Again, if you're modeling your menu after the Finish Strong phase (Days 15 to 21) or are eating to maintain your loss, you can add a ½-cup serving of couscous or brown rice or 2 ounces of whole-grain bread.

> ▶ **Orange Beef with Green Beans, Broccoli & Bok Choy** (page 188)
> ▶ **Southwestern Chile Verde** (page 182)
> ▶ **Quinoa Fritters with Spicy Pepper Sauce** (page 200)
> ▶ **Meatballs & Spaghetti Squash** (page 185)

After a few days of mixing and matching according to these rules, you'll get the hang of it—I promise! I'm also a big fan of learning by doing. By the end of the 21-Day Plan, you should be able to eyeball a plate and make an educated guess as to whether it contains proper portions and a healthy mix of protein, fat, and carbs.

You'll also learn how to adapt recipes to your tastes by discovering which fat releasers are your favorites. Our test team became quite versatile in the kitchen, substituting chicken for turkey or adding a bit more vinegar to sauces if that's what their taste buds called for. And that's the best way to stick to any diet for life—to find small ways to make it yours.

● RECIPES FOR THE REAL WORLD

In my 20+ years as a health journalist, I've learned that the number one barrier to healthy eating is taste. People wrongfully equate "healthy" with "bland" and "uninviting." That's why I was so gratified to hear the daily feedback from the test team: Folks like Joe Rinaldi gushing about Day 9's menu: "Two thumbs up for breakfast. Never thought to put fat-free cream cheese on eggs!" Or Margaret Jones, who said of the Grilled Turkey Cutlets with Lemon and Marjoram (page 183): "So delicious—so happy I have extra for another night this week." We got raves about the shakes, soups, dinners, and more.

I'm not telling you this to brag—I tell you with the intention of busting the myth that healthy food doesn't taste good. It was important to me that our recipes pass this real-world "taste test." The test team's reaction confirmed that healthy food is delicious and crave-worthy. We don't have to "settle" or deprive ourselves to take care of our bodies.

I've been waiting all book long to say this: Let's get cooking!

Strawberry Almond Shake

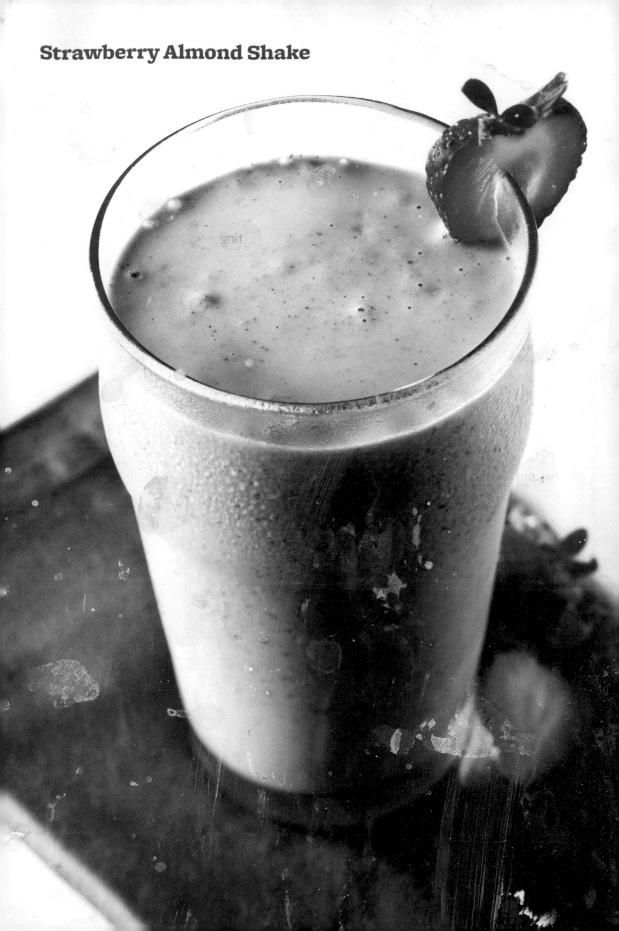

Fast Release Shake (Days 1–4)

Hands-On Time: 10 minutes • **Total Time:** 10 minutes • **Makes:** 1 shake

Pick your favorite shake and stick with it for simplicity, or if you're feeling adventurous, plan a different flavor combination for every day. Remember, during this stage of the diet, you'll be drinking two shakes a day (see Chapter 4, pages 85–90). Note that the shake is minimally sweet on purpose to keep you from getting hungry too soon. Please don't be tempted to add more honey.

Fat Releasers
Yogurt, coconut milk, fruit/fiber, healthy fats, honey

MASTER RECIPE

¾ cup (6 ounces) nonfat yogurt

¼ cup light coconut milk

3 tablespoons nonfat milk powder

FRUIT/FIBER

HEALTHY FATS

2 teaspoons honey

½ teaspoon vanilla extract

FLAVORINGS (optional)

4 ice cubes

Combine all the ingredients in a blender and blend until nice and frothy.

A typical shake:

- 395 calories • 16g protein
- 18g fat (5g saturated)
- 9.5g fiber • 430mg calcium
- 40mg vitamin C
- 50g carbohydrate
- 210mg sodium

FRUIT/FIBER (choose 1)

1 banana

1 apple (peeled and cored) + 1 tablespoon flaxseed meal

8 strawberries (fresh or frozen) + 1 tablespoon flaxseed meal

4 ounces mixed frozen berries* (¾ to 1 cup, depending on the berries' size) + 1 tablespoon flaxseed meal

¾ cup seedless red grapes* (10 large) + 1 tablespoon flaxseed meal. Omit the honey.

1 tangerine or small orange* + 1 tablespoon flaxseed meal

HEALTHY FATS (choose 1)

½ avocado

1 tablespoon natural peanut butter

1 tablespoon raw or regular almond butter

1 tablespoon tahini

1 tablespoon sunflower seed butter

FLAVORINGS (choose none, 1, or both)

1 teaspoon unsweetened cocoa powder

¼ teaspoon ground cinnamon

*See Tasty Tips, page 154.

Peanut Butter and Grape Shake

Tasty Tips

▶ In the grape version, you can first wash and dry individual grapes, then freeze them. Add them to the blender frozen.

▶ If the berry mix includes blackberries, be prepared for their seeds (which are a good source of fiber).

▶ The tangerine/ orange version tastes like a creamsicle, but you have to cut the segments out from between the membranes or you get big pieces of skin in the shake.

Fade Away Shake (Days 5–14)

Hands-On Time: 10 minutes • **Total Time:** 10 minutes • **Makes:** 1 shake

This is principally the same as the Fast Release Shake (page 153), but the amount of fat has been cut back, since the focus in this phase is on lean protein and including more macronutrients in your meals. Remember, at this stage, you will be drinking a shake once a day, while snacking twice a day. To refresh: See Chapter 4, pages 90–92.

Fat Releasers
Yogurt, coconut milk, fruit/fiber, healthy fats, honey

MASTER RECIPE

- ¾ cup (6 ounces) nonfat yogurt
- 2 tablespoons light coconut milk
- 2 tablespoons water
- 3 tablespoons nonfat milk powder
- FRUIT/FIBER
- HEALTHY FATS
- 2 teaspoons honey
- ½ teaspoon vanilla extract
- FLAVORINGS (optional)
- 4 ice cubes

Combine all the ingredients in a blender and blend until nice and frothy.

A typical shake:
- 320 calories • 15g protein
- 11g fat (2.5g saturated)
- 7g fiber • 425mg calcium
- 40mg vitamin C
- 45g carbohydrate
- 205mg sodium

FRUIT/FIBER (choose 1)

1 banana

1 apple (peeled and cored) + 1 tablespoon flaxseed meal

8 strawberries (fresh or frozen) + 1 tablespoon flaxseed meal

4 ounces mixed frozen berries* (¾ to 1 cup, depending on the berries' size) + 1 tablespoon flaxseed meal

¾ cup seedless red grapes* (10 large) + 1 tablespoon flaxseed meal. Omit the honey.

1 tangerine or small orange* + 1 tablespoon flaxseed meal

HEALTHY FATS (choose 1)

¼ avocado

1 teaspoon natural peanut butter

1 teaspoon raw or regular almond butter

1 teaspoon tahini

1 teaspoon sunflower seed butter

FLAVORINGS (choose none, 1, or both)

1 teaspoon unsweetened cocoa powder

¼ teaspoon ground cinnamon

*See Tasty Tips, opposite.

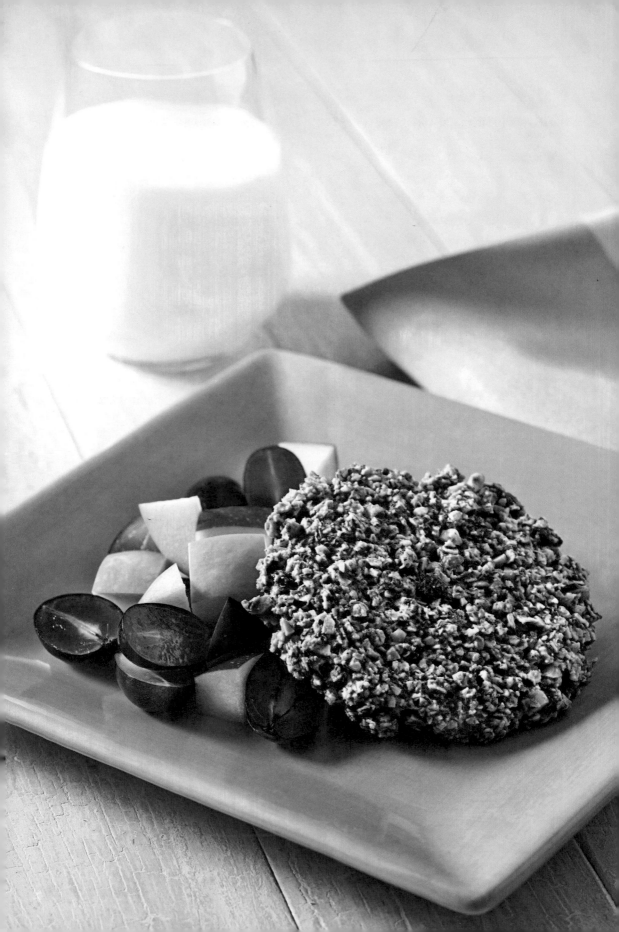

Oatmeal Breakfast Cakes

Hands-On Time: 20 minutes • **Total Time:** 30 minutes • **Makes:** 8 servings

An oatmeal cake is the perfect solution for someone who wants to have that bowl of oatmeal but is always on the go. These breakfast cakes are great to freeze; just pop them in the toaster oven or the microwave to warm them up. Have them with a serving of dairy and some fruit on top.

Fat Releasers
Oats, nuts, honey, flaxseed, yogurt, olive oil, egg

1½ cups quick-cooking oats

¼ cup (1 ounce) finely chopped nuts/seeds (see Options below)

¼ cup flaxseed meal

½ teaspoon baking soda

¼ teaspoon fine sea salt

3 tablespoons chopped dates (about 5 dates)

¼ cup + 2 tablespoons nonfat yogurt

2 tablespoons extra-light olive oil

2 tablespoons honey

1 egg

▶ **NUT/SEED OPTIONS:** Spanish peanuts (good source of resveratrol), regular peanuts, walnuts, almonds, pecans, pistachios, cashews, sunflower seeds, pumpkin seeds

1. Preheat the oven to 350°F. Line a baking sheet with parchment paper or a nonstick liner.

2. In a large bowl, stir together the oats, nuts/seeds, flaxseed meal, baking soda, and salt until very well combined. Work in the dates with your hands, separating the clumps and making sure they're evenly distributed.

3. Make a well in the center of the oat mixture and add the yogurt, oil, honey, and egg. Beat the wet ingredients together with a fork, then start stirring in the oat mixture to form a wet dough.

4. With a ¼-cup measure, scoop out the dough and plop 1 inch apart on the baking sheet (you should get 8 cakes). With wet hands, pat the dough into even cakes about ½ inch high. Bake until lightly golden but still nice and soft, 16 to 18 minutes.

5. Let cool on the baking sheet for 2 minutes, then transfer to a wire rack to cool completely. Store them in the fridge or the freezer.

Per 1-cake serving: 177 calories • 5g protein • 8.5g fat (1g saturated) • 3.5g fiber 54mg calcium • 0mg vitamin C • 21g carbohydrate • 171mg sodium

Full-of-Options Omelets

Hands-On Time: 10 minutes • **Total Time:** 10 minutes • **Makes:** 1 serving

If you prefer to use egg substitute, you'll need ½ cup. Or, for an all-egg-white omelet, use 4 egg whites (or ½ cup liquid egg whites). See the options below for ways to vary the flavor of this omelet.

Fat Releasers
Eggs, milk, black pepper

- 1 **large egg**
- 2 **large egg whites**
- 1 **tablespoon fat-free or 1% milk**
- **Sea salt and black pepper**

1. In a small bowl, combine the egg, egg whites, milk, and salt and pepper to taste. Whisk well until just slightly frothy.

2. Spray a medium (10-inch) nonstick skillet with olive oil and heat over medium heat. Pour in the egg mixture and, as it cooks, pull it away from the sides of the pan to let the uncooked egg flow underneath. After 1 to 2 minutes, cover and cook until the top is set and the bottom is nicely browned, about 1 minute.

3. Remove from the heat. Fold the omelet in half and slide out of the pan.

Per serving: 125 calories • 14g protein • 6.5g fat (1.5g saturated) • 0g fiber 52mg calcium • 0mg vitamin C • 2g carbohydrate • 257mg sodium

▶ OMELET OPTIONS

Mexilicious: Add a pinch of ground cumin and ½ teaspoon minced red or green serrano chiles, if desired, to the egg mixture. After removing from the heat, top with 2 tablespoons shredded reduced-fat cheddar cheese and 2 tablespoons chopped fresh cilantro.
Per serving: 165 calories• 17g protein• 9.5g fat (3.5g saturated)• 0g fiber 252mg calcium• 0mg vitamin C• 2g carbohydrate• 372mg sodium

California Dream: After removing from the heat, top with ¼ small thinly sliced avocado, 1 chopped artichoke heart (water-packed), and 2 teaspoons shredded Parmesan cheese.
Per serving: 203 calories• 16g protein• 12g fat (3g saturated)• 3g fiber 98mg calcium• 5mg vitamin C• 6g carbohydrate• 400mg sodium

Creamy Quinoa

Hands-On Time: 10 minutes • **Total Time:** 20 minutes • **Makes:** 4 servings

Quinoa is a grain that contains high-quality protein, so it's a really good way to start the day. And cooking it with milk adds more protein and lots of calcium. If you make the whole batch ahead and refrigerate it, you can have hot cereal at a moment's notice. Just scoop out ½ cup, place it in a bowl with a little fat-free milk, and microwave it on high for about 45 seconds. Then top with the honey and nuts. If you're on the last week of the diet, you can add cut-up fruit.

Fat Releasers
Quinoa, milk, flaxseed, honey, nuts

---

1 **cup quinoa**
Generous pinch of fine sea
   salt
1½ **cups water**
1 **cup fat-free evaporated**
   milk
2 **tablespoons flaxseed meal**
4 **teaspoons honey**
1 **teaspoon vanilla extract**
   or ½ teaspoon almond
   extract
1 **cup fat-free milk**
8 **teaspoons chopped nuts/**
   seeds (see Options below)

▶ **NUT/SEED OPTIONS:** Spanish peanuts (good source of resveratrol), regular peanuts, walnuts, almonds, pecans, pistachios, cashews, sunflower seeds, pumpkin seeds

1. In a medium saucepan, combine the quinoa, salt, and water. Bring to a boil. Reduce to a simmer, cover, and cook for 10 minutes (the quinoa should be tender, but it's okay if it's still a little wet).

2. Uncover, stir in the evaporated milk, flaxseed meal, and 2 teaspoons of the honey. Return to a simmer and cook, stirring, until the milk is mostly absorbed and the cereal is a thickness you like, 4 to 6 minutes.

3. Remove from the heat and stir in the vanilla or almond extract. Top each serving with ¼ cup milk, ½ teaspoon honey, and 2 teaspoons chopped nuts/seeds.

Per ¾-cup serving: 286 calories • 14g protein • 5.5g fat (0.5g saturated) • 4.5g fiber 289mg calcium • 1mg vitamin C • 45g carbohydrate • 154mg sodium

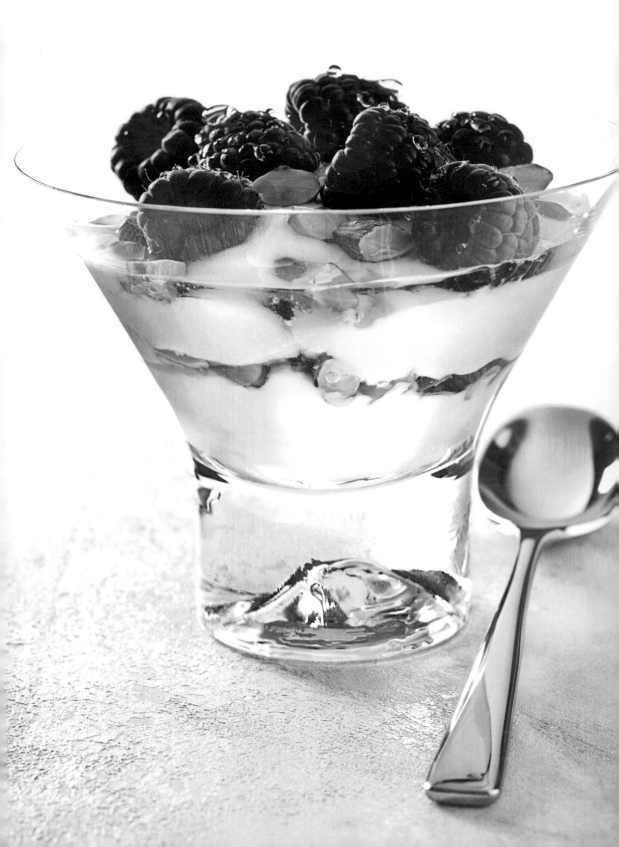

Honey-Nut Yogurt Parfait

Hands-On Time: 10 minutes • **Total Time:** 10 minutes • **Makes:** 4 servings

This glamorous parfait really makes you look forward to breakfast: It's so creamy and luscious, it hardly seems legal! You can swap out the berries and add sliced peaches or nectarines or a mixture of fruits instead.

Fat Releasers
Yogurt, almonds, honey, raspberries

2⅔ cups 0% Greek yogurt

8 tablespoons chopped toasted almonds

2 cups raspberries

8 teaspoons honey

Put ⅓ cup of the yogurt into each of four 8-ounce glasses or bowls. Add 1 tablespoon of the almonds and ¼ cup of the raspberries, then drizzle with 1 teaspoon of the honey. Repeat the layering with the remaining ingredients.

Per serving (1 parfait): 232 calories • 17g protein • 7g fat (0.5g saturated) 5.7g fiber • 152mg calcium • 16mg vitamin C • 28g carbohydrate • 58mg sodium

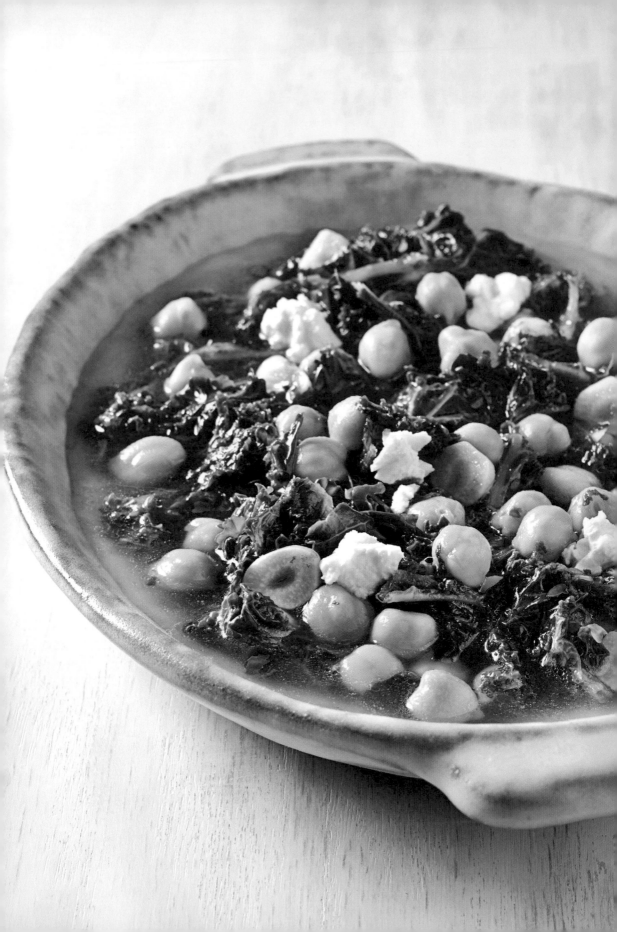

Kale & Chickpea Soup with Feta Cheese

Hands-On Time: 20 minutes • **Total Time:** 40 minutes • **Makes:** 8 cups

This hearty combination of kale and chickpeas is a variation on the Portuguese soup, caldo verde. Typically, the soup's flavor is brightened with vinegar, which luckily is also a fat releaser. If you want to freeze the soup, leave out the cheese and add it when you reheat. To add a little more protein, you can poach eggs in the simmering soup just before serving.

Fat Releasers
Garlic, red pepper flakes, olive oil, kale, chickpeas, black pepper, vinegar, feta cheese

- 6 **large cloves garlic, thinly sliced**
- ½ **teaspoon red pepper flakes**
- 2 **tablespoons extra-virgin olive oil**
- 1 **pound kale, center ribs discarded, leaves finely chopped (8 cups)**
- 3 **cups low-sodium chicken broth**
- 3 **cups water**
- 2 **cans (15 ounces each) no-salt-added chickpeas, rinsed and drained**
- ½ **teaspoon black pepper**
- 2 **tablespoons red-wine vinegar**
- ¼ **cup (1½ ounces) crumbled reduced-fat feta cheese**

1. In a 5- to 6-quart pot, cook the garlic and pepper flakes in the oil over medium heat, stirring occasionally, just until the garlic begins to color, about 3 minutes. Stir in the kale and cook, stirring frequently, until wilted, about 5 minutes.

2. Add the broth, water, chickpeas, and black pepper. Cover and simmer until the kale is very tender, about 20 minutes.

3. Stir in the vinegar. Sprinkle each serving with ½ tablespoon feta cheese.

Per 1-cup serving: 172 calories • 9g protein • 5g fat (1g saturated) • 5.5g fiber 110mg calcium • 25mg vitamin C • 24g carbohydrate • 124mg sodium

Per 2-cup serving: 344 calories • 17g protein • 10g fat (2g saturated) • 11g fiber 219mg calcium • 50mg vitamin C • 47g carbohydrate • 248mg sodium

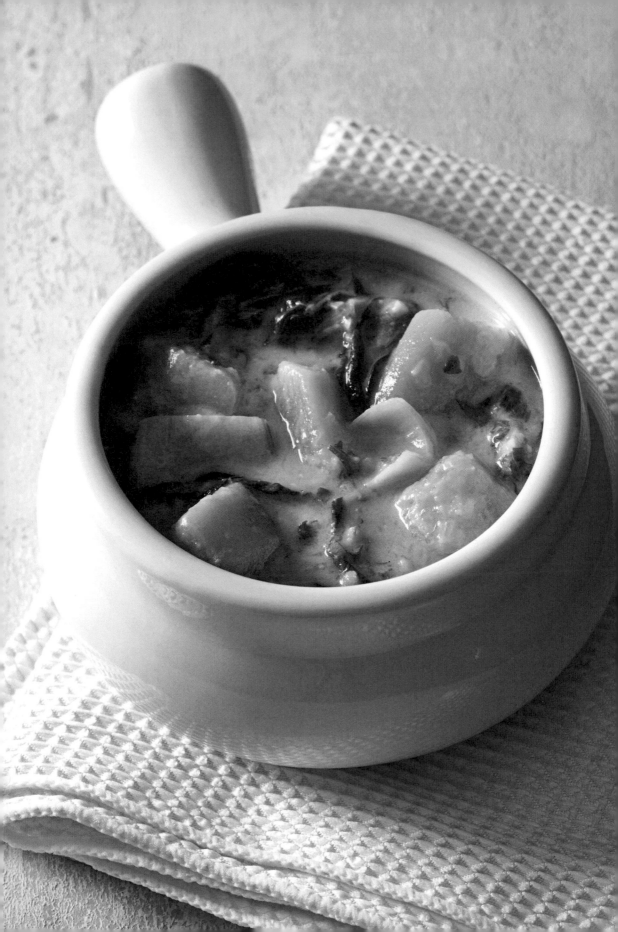

Spiced Winter Squash Soup with Asian Greens

Hands-On Time: 10 minutes • **Total Time:** 35 minutes • **Makes:** 10 cups

This soup is easy to do when you start with frozen winter squash. This recipe makes enough for the first four days of the diet, with 2 cups left over. Freeze them in 1-cup containers and have a bowl for lunch in place of any of the suggested lunches.

Fat Releasers
Squash, coconut milk, lentils, peanut butter, garlic, ginger, red pepper flakes, bok choy, scallions, lime

- 2 packages (10 ounces each) frozen cubed or mashed winter squash, thawed
- 4 cups low-sodium chicken broth
- 1 cup light coconut milk
- 1 cup red lentils
- ¼ cup natural peanut butter
- 2 cloves garlic, finely chopped
- 2-inch piece fresh ginger, peeled and minced
- ½ teaspoon red pepper flakes
- ¾ pound Asian greens, such as baby bok choy or tatsoi, cut into 1-inch pieces (5 cups packed)
- ¼ cup chopped scallions
- ¼ cup chopped fresh cilantro
- 2 tablespoons fresh lime juice

1. In a 5- to 6-quart pot, combine the squash, broth, coconut milk, lentils, peanut butter, garlic, ginger, and pepper flakes. Bring to a simmer over medium heat, cover, and cook, stirring occasionally, until the lentils are tender, about 20 minutes.

2. Add the greens and simmer until wilted, about 5 minutes. Stir in the scallions, cilantro, and lime juice.

Per 1-cup serving: 168 calories • 9g protein • 5g fat (1.5g saturated) • 4.5g fiber 65mg calcium • 20mg vitamin C • 24g carbohydrate • 57mg sodium

Per 2-cup serving: 335 calories • 18g protein • 10g fat (3g saturated) • 9g fiber 130mg calcium • 39mg vitamin C • 47g carbohydrate • 115mg sodium

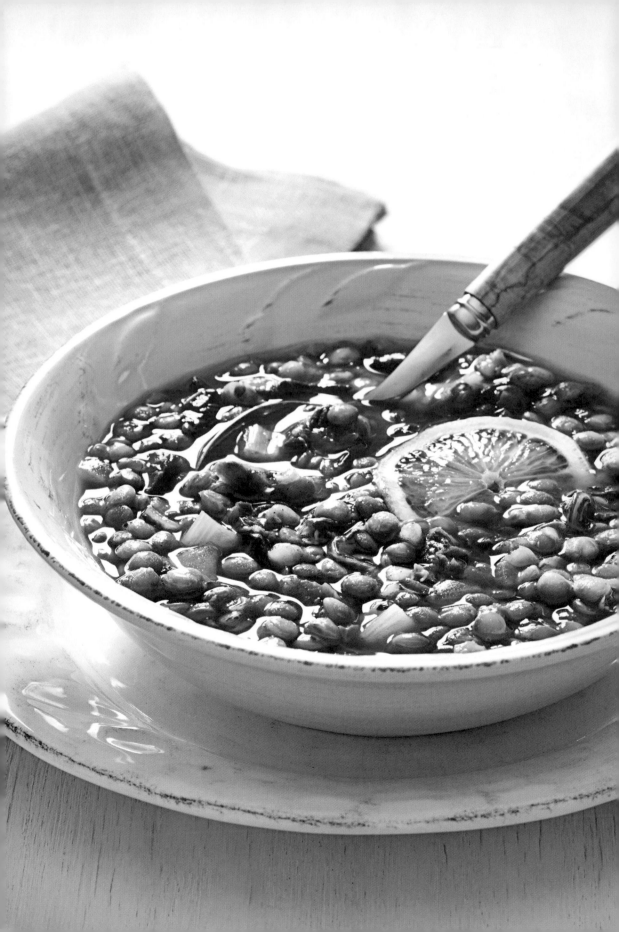

Lemony Lentil & Chard Soup

Hands-On Time: 20 minutes • **Total Time:** 50 minutes • **Makes:** 12 cups

Garnish the soup with a thin slice of lemon. Spinach is a good substitute for the chard. This recipe makes enough for the first four days of the diet, with 4 cups left over. Freeze them in 1-cup containers and have a bowl at lunch in place of any of the suggested lunches.

Fat Releasers
Olive oil, onion, garlic, lentils, lemon, sun-dried tomatoes, black pepper

- 1 **pound green Swiss chard**
- 2 **tablespoons extra-virgin olive oil**
- 1 **large onion, chopped**
- 3 **cloves garlic, chopped**
- 1 **bay leaf**
- 7 **cups water**
- 2 **cups dried lentils**
- ¼ **cup fresh lemon juice**
- ¼ **cup chopped dry-pack sun-dried tomatoes**
- ½ **teaspoon ground allspice**
- ½ **teaspoon coarse sea salt**
- ½ **teaspoon black pepper**

1. Separate the leaves and center ribs of the chard. Chop the ribs into ½-inch pieces (2 cups). Coarsely chop the leaves (about 8 cups packed).

2. In a 5- to 6-quart pot, heat the oil over medium heat. Add the chard ribs, onion, garlic, and bay leaf and cook, stirring occasionally, until softened and beginning to brown, about 10 minutes.

3. Add the water, chard leaves, lentils, lemon juice, tomatoes, allspice, salt, and pepper. Cover and simmer until the lentils and chard are very tender, about 30 minutes. Discard bay leaf.

Per 1-cup serving: 151 calories • 9g protein • 2.5g fat (0.5g saturated) • 11g fiber 44mg calcium • 16mg vitamin C • 23g carbohydrate • 187mg sodium

Per 2-cup serving: 301 calories • 19g protein • 5.5g fat (1g saturated) • 22g fiber 88mg calcium • 33mg vitamin C • 46g carbohydrate • 374mg sodium

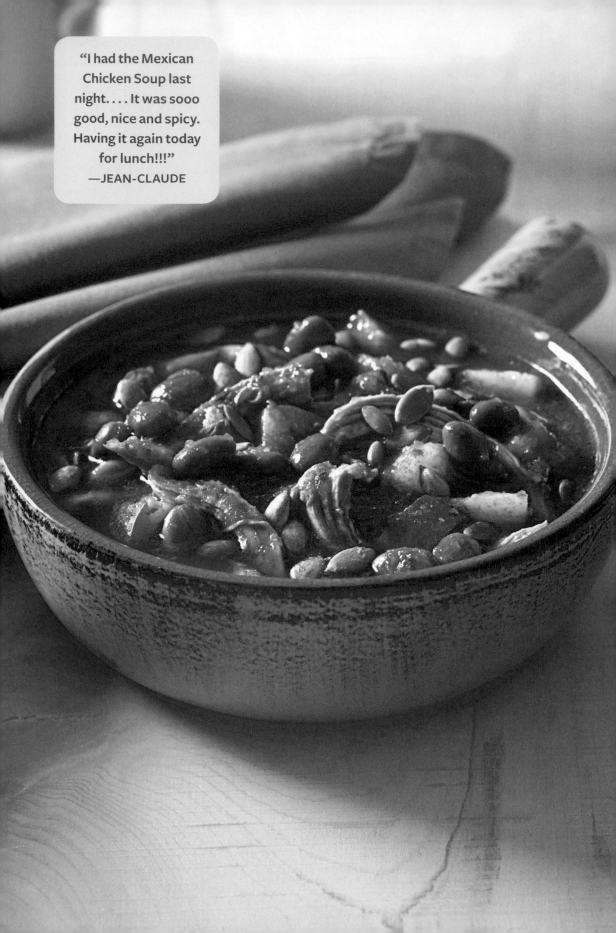

"I had the Mexican Chicken Soup last night. . . . It was sooo good, nice and spicy. Having it again today for lunch!!!"
—JEAN-CLAUDE

Hearty Mexican Chicken Soup

Hands-On Time: 25 minutes • **Total Time:** 1 hour • **Makes:** 10 cups

This recipe makes enough for the first four days of the diet, with 2 cups left over. Freeze them in 1-cup containers and have a bowl for lunch in place of any of the suggested lunches.

Fat Releasers
Peppers, onion, garlic, oregano, chicken, olive oil, zucchini, beans, lime, seeds

4 dried ancho chiles, wiped with a damp cloth

2 cups boiling water

4 cups low-sodium chicken broth

1 pound skinless, boneless chicken breasts

1 onion, chopped

2 cloves garlic, chopped

1½ teaspoons dried oregano

¼ teaspoon black pepper

2 tablespoons olive oil

1 pound zucchini, cut into ½-inch pieces (3 cups)

1 can (15 ounces) no-salt-added pinto beans, rinsed and drained

¼ teaspoon coarse sea salt

1 tablespoon fresh lime juice

¼ cup hulled pumpkin seeds, toasted

1. In a heatproof bowl, combine the chiles and water. Let soak about 30 minutes. Reserve the soaking liquid.

2. Bring the broth to a simmer in a 2-quart saucepan. Add the chicken and simmer gently, covered, until the chicken is just cooked through, about 15 minutes. Transfer the chicken to a bowl with a slotted spoon and let cool; shred. Reserve broth.

3. Stem and seed the chiles and transfer to a blender. Add the reserved soaking liquid, onion, garlic, oregano, and pepper. Puree until smooth.

4. In a 5-quart pot, heat the oil over medium heat until it shimmers, then carefully add the chile puree (it will splatter) and cook, stirring frequently, until thickened, about 10 minutes. Add the reserved broth, zucchini, and beans and simmer, covered, until the zucchini is tender, about 10 minutes.

5. Stir in the chicken, salt, and lime juice and simmer, just until the chicken is heated, about 2 minutes. Top each serving with a generous teaspoon of pumpkin seeds.

Per 1-cup serving: 174 calories • 15g protein • 7g fat (1g saturated) • 4.5g fiber 42mg calcium • 10mg vitamin C • 13g carbohydrate • 141mg sodium

Per 2-cup serving: 349 calories • 31g protein • 14g fat (2.5g saturated) • 9g fiber 84mg calcium • 21mg vitamin C • 26g carbohydrate • 282mg sodium

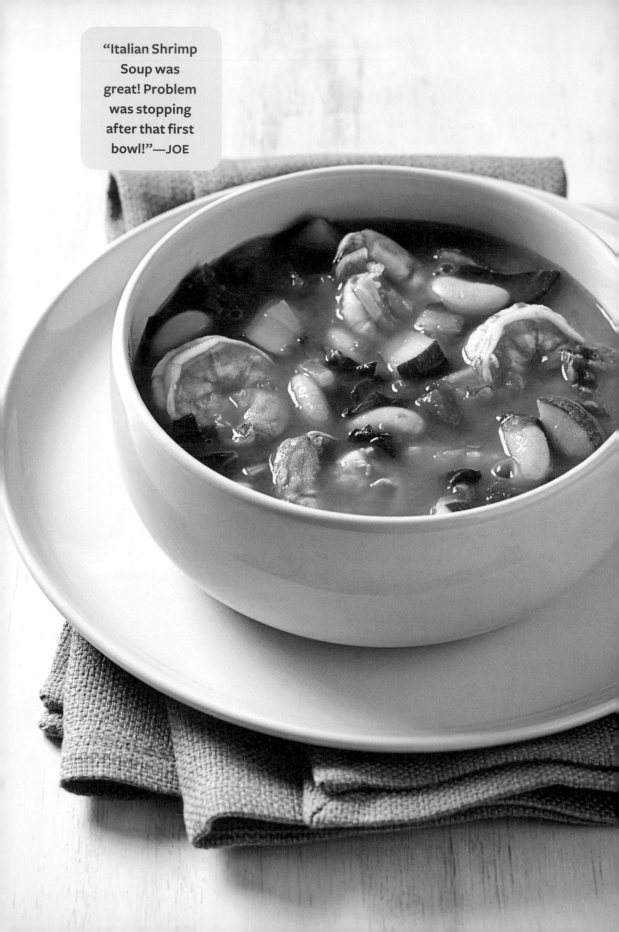

"Italian Shrimp Soup was great! Problem was stopping after that first bowl!" —JOE

Italian Shrimp & Vegetable Soup

Hands-On Time: 35 minutes • **Total Time:** 1 hour 10 minutes • **Makes:** 14 cups

Although this Italian-inspired soup makes quite a large batch, it is so low in calories that you can have a 2-cup serving anytime. It will freeze well, but be sure to reheat it gently so the shrimp will remain tender.

Fat Releasers
Onion, marjoram, red pepper flakes, garlic, zucchini, olive oil, escarole, tomatoes, beans, shrimp

- 1 large fennel bulb, stalks discarded, bulb chopped (3 cups)
- 1 onion, chopped
- 2 celery stalks, chopped
- 3 cloves garlic, chopped
- 2 tablespoons extra-virgin olive oil
- 1 teaspoon dried marjoram
- ½ teaspoon hot red pepper flakes
- ¼ teaspoon coarse sea salt
- 1 pound zucchini, cut into 1-inch pieces
- 1 head escarole (1 pound), coarsely chopped
- 5 cups water
- 1 can (14.5 ounces) no-salt-added diced tomatoes
- 1 pound peeled and deveined medium shrimp
- 1 can (15 ounces) no-salt-added white beans, such as cannellini or Great Northern, rinsed and drained

1. In a 5- to 6-quart pot over medium heat, cook the fennel, onion, celery, and garlic in the oil with the marjoram, pepper flakes, and salt, stirring occasionally, until the vegetables are softened and beginning to brown, about 15 minutes.

2. Stir in the zucchini and escarole and cook, stirring occasionally, until the escarole is wilted, about 10 minutes. Add the water and tomatoes (with juice) and simmer, covered, until the vegetables are tender, about 10 minutes.

3. Stir in the shrimp and beans and gently simmer, uncovered, just until the shrimp are cooked through, about 2 minutes.

Per 2-cup serving: 193 calories • 15g protein • 5.5g fat (0.5g saturated) • 8g fiber 151mg calcium • 35mg vitamin C • 23g carbohydrate • 524mg sodium

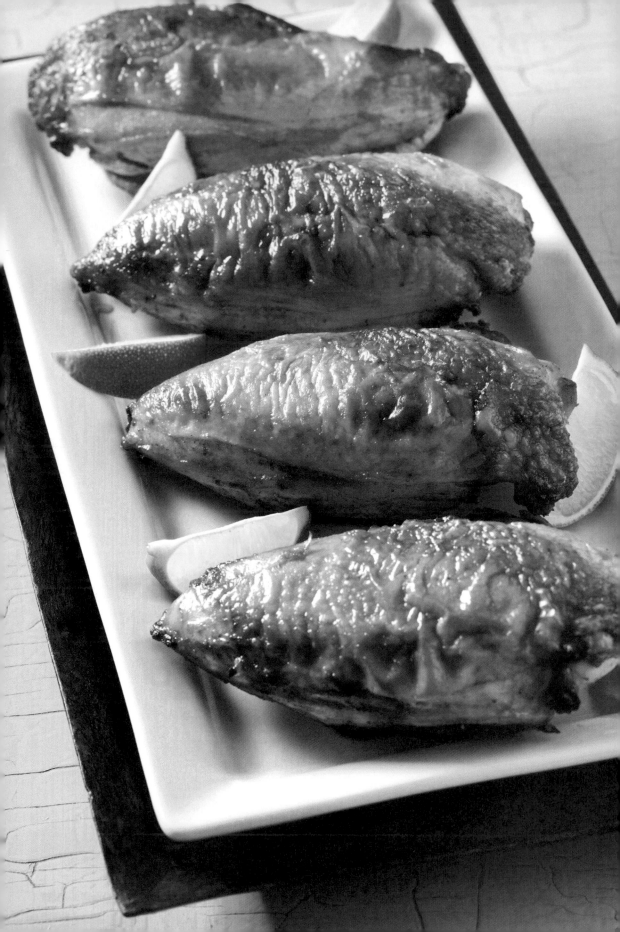

Big-Batch Roast Chicken

Hands-On Time: 10 minutes • **Total Time:** 50 minutes • **Makes:** 8 servings

Here's an idea: Do a mix-and-match. Make up a couple of different seasoning mixtures and roast all the chicken in the same pan. That way, you'll have many choices throughout the week. To plan for leftovers: You can cook anywhere from 1 to 8 breasts according to these directions, depending on how many you need for dinner, and how many you want to save for later in the week. Store extra chicken with the skin on until you're ready to eat it.

Fat Releaser
Chicken

8   **bone-in, skin-on chicken breast halves (about 8 ounces each)**
SEASONING (see next page)

1. In a large bowl, mix up SEASONING. Add the chicken to the bowl and rub the SEASONING all over any exposed portions of flesh and under the skin (don't waste any seasoning on top of the skin, because it will be discarded; the skin just stays on during roasting to help keep the chicken moist). Let the chicken sit in the bowl while the oven preheats.
2. Preheat the oven to 400°F.
3. Arrange the chicken, skin-side up, on a large-rimmed baking sheet and roast until the juices run clear and the chicken is cooked through but still moist, 30 to 35 minutes. Remove from the oven and let rest for 10 minutes before serving. Remove the skin before eating.

Per serving: 105 calories • 20g protein • 2.5g fat (0.5g saturated) • 0g fiber 10mg calcium • 0mg vitamin C • 0g carbohydrate • 47mg sodium

▶ SEASONINGS: Big-Batch Roast Chicken

Lemon–Garlic: 5 grated garlic cloves (use a citrus zester), ¼ cup fresh lemon juice, and ½ teaspoon black pepper
Fat Releasers: Garlic, lemon, black pepper
Per serving: 110 calories• 20g protein• 2.5g fat (0.5g saturated) • 0g fiber
14mg calcium• 4mg vitamin C• 1g carbohydrate• 48mg sodium

Chili–Lime: 1 tablespoon + 1 teaspoon chili powder, grated zest of 1 lime, and juice of 2 limes
Fat Releasers: Chili powder, lime
Per serving: 107 calories• 20g protein• 2.5g fat (0.5g saturated) • 0g fiber
11mg calcium• 3mg vitamin C• 1g carbohydrate• 47mg sodium

Moroccan: ¼ cup water, 1 tablespoon olive oil, 1 tablespoon + 1 teaspoon ground cumin, 2 teaspoons ground cinnamon, ½ teaspoon fine sea salt, and ½ teaspoon black pepper
Fat Releasers: Olive oil, cinnamon, black pepper
Per serving: 125 calories• 20g protein• 4g fat (1g saturated) • 0.5g fiber
18mg calcium• 0mg vitamin C• 0g carbohydrate• 195mg sodium

Smoked Paprika: ¼ cup + 2 tablespoons balsamic vinegar and 1 tablespoon + 1 teaspoon smoked paprika
Fat Releaser: Vinegar
Per serving: 120 calories• 20g protein• 2.5g fat (0.5g saturated) • 0.5g fiber
15mg calcium• 0mg vitamin C• 3g carbohydrate• 51mg sodium

Poached Chicken with Garlic-Walnut Sauce

Hands-On Time: 15 minutes ● **Total Time:** 40 minutes ● **Makes:** 4 servings

This recipe's herbal walnut sauce is scrumptious not only on chicken but also on steamed green beans or broccoli. Any leftover chicken and sauce will make a tasty sandwich when tossed with baby arugula and rolled up in a high-fiber wrap (see pages 116–117). Save the broth from step 1 for a quick soup: Combine the broth, cooked beans (page 222), no-salt-added diced tomatoes, and baby spinach. Season to taste with a Fat Releaser Seasoning (page 111).

Fat Releasers
Chicken, garlic, cayenne pepper, walnuts, parsley, lemons

- 4 **cups low-sodium chicken broth**
- 1 **pound skinless, boneless chicken breasts**
- 1 **small clove garlic**
- ⅛ **teaspoon fine sea salt**
- ¼ **teaspoon cayenne pepper**
- ¼ **cup chopped toasted walnuts**
- 2½ **tablespoons chopped flat-leaf parsley**
- 2½ **tablespoons chopped fresh cilantro**
- ½ **teaspoon fresh lemon juice**

1. In a 2-quart saucepan, bring the stock to a simmer. Add the chicken, cover, and simmer gently until the chicken is just cooked through, about 15 minutes. With a slotted spoon, transfer the chicken to a bowl and keep warm. Reserve ⅓ cup of the broth, and save the remaining broth for another use.

2. Mince and mash the garlic with the salt to a paste using the side of a heavy knife. Transfer the paste to a blender with the cayenne, walnuts, 2 tablespoons of the parsley, 2 tablespoons of the cilantro, the lemon juice, and the reserved broth. Puree the sauce until smooth.

3. Slice the chicken and serve drizzled with the walnut sauce and sprinkled with the remaining parsley and cilantro.

Per serving: 183 calories ● 26g protein ● 8g fat (1g saturated) ● 0.5g fiber 18mg calcium ● 5mg vitamin C ● 2g carbohydrate ● 223mg sodium

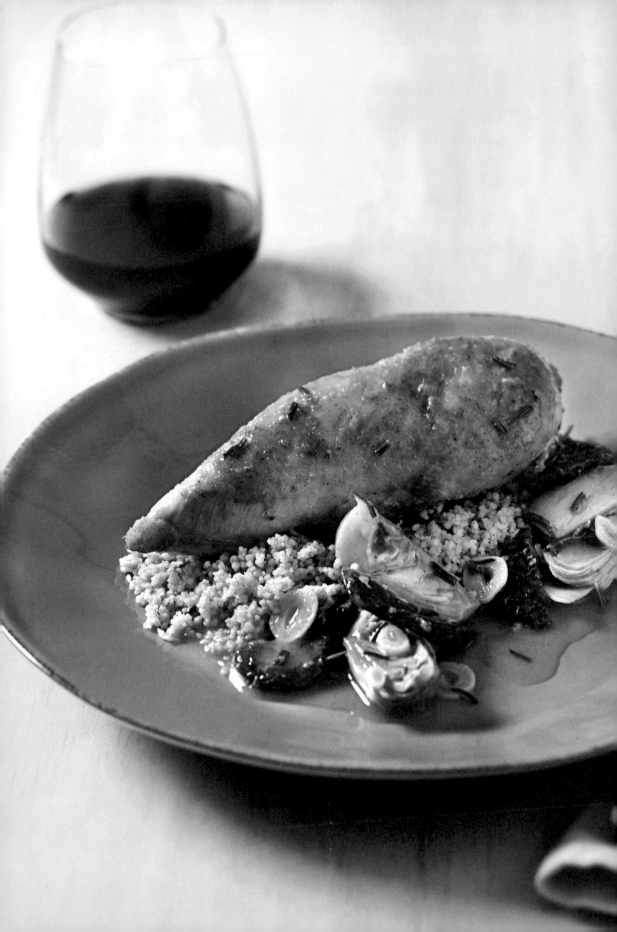

Braised Chicken with Artichokes & Sun-Dried Tomatoes

Hands-On Time: 15 minutes ● **Total Time:** 25 minutes ● **Makes:** 4 servings

If you've moved past the Fade Away portion of the diet and are in Finish Strong, you can serve the chicken with whole-wheat couscous (page 227) or brown rice (pages 228–229).

Fat Releasers
Olive oil, chicken, garlic, artichokes, tomatoes, orange, rosemary, black pepper

1 tablespoon extra-virgin olive oil

4 skinless, bone-in chicken breast halves (about 6 ounces each)

2 tablespoons whole-wheat flour

3 cloves garlic, thinly sliced

1 cup low-sodium chicken broth

1 package (9 ounces) frozen artichoke hearts, thawed and quartered

⅓ cup dry-pack sun-dried tomatoes, thinly sliced

½ teaspoon grated orange zest

¼ cup fresh orange juice

½ teaspoon chopped fresh or dried rosemary

½ teaspoon fine sea salt

¼ teaspoon black pepper

1. In a large skillet, heat the oil over medium-high heat. Dredge the chicken in the flour, add to the pan, and cook until golden brown on both sides, about 5 minutes. Transfer to a plate.

2. Reduce the heat to medium, add the garlic to the pan and cook until golden brown, about 2 minutes.

3. Add the broth, artichokes, tomatoes, orange zest, orange juice, rosemary, salt, and pepper and bring to a boil.

4. Return the chicken to the pan and reduce to a simmer. Cover and cook until the chicken is cooked through, about 5 minutes.

Per serving: 247 calories ● 31g protein ● 7.5g fat (1.5g saturated) ● 5g fiber 57mg calcium ● 14mg vitamin C ● 13g carbohydrate ● 366mg sodium

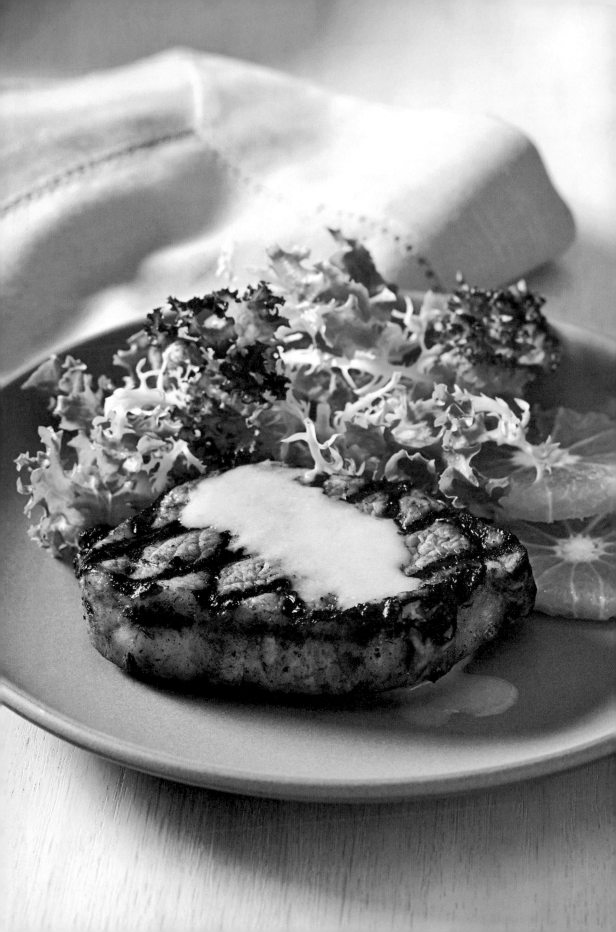

Citrus- & Herb-Marinated Pork Chops

Hands-On Time: 10 minutes • **Total Time:** 1 hour 15 minutes • **Makes:** 4 servings

For convenience, you can assemble the marinade and pork in the morning and let it marinate in the fridge until ready to cook. Or if you happen to have a vacuum-style marinator, you can make this dish last minute and marinate for only 5 to 10 minutes. This marinade also works really well with chicken. The mustard-orange sauce, which is light and made without any oil, could be used to dress a dish of simple steamed spinach or green beans.

Fat Releasers
Orange, lemon, lime, garlic, thyme, black pepper, pork, olive oil

¼ cup + 2 tablespoons fresh orange juice

1 tablespoon fresh lemon juice

1 tablespoon fresh lime juice

2 cloves garlic, smashed

½ teaspoon dried thyme

½ teaspoon dried sage

½ teaspoon fine sea salt

¼ teaspoon black pepper

4 boneless loin pork chops (5 ounces each), well trimmed

1 tablespoon Dijon mustard

1 tablespoon + 1 teaspoon olive oil

1. In a large plastic resealable bag, combine 2 tablespoons of the orange juice, the lemon juice, lime juice, garlic, thyme, sage, salt, and pepper. Add the pork to the bag and seal tightly before shaking it to evenly coat the meat. Marinate for at least 1 hour and up to 8 hours in the refrigerator.

2. In a small bowl, whisk together the mustard and remaining ¼ cup orange juice. Set aside.

3. Brush a grill pan with the oil and preheat. Add the pork and grill for 4 minutes on the first side. Flip and grill the other side until cooked through but still juicy, about 2 minutes longer.

4. Serve the pork with the mustard sauce.

Per serving: 248 calories • 27g protein • 14g fat (4g saturated) • 0g fiber
34mg calcium • 10mg vitamin C • 3g carbohydrate • 294mg sodium

Turkey-Mushroom Burgers

Hands-On Time: 10 minutes • **Total Time:** 20 minutes • **Makes:** 4 servings

These burgers freeze beautifully. Make the patties (through step 2) and wrap them separately in plastic and then in foil to prevent freezer burn. Defrost overnight in the refrigerator before cooking.

Fat Releasers
Yogurt, garlic, turkey, black pepper, tomatoes

- 8 ounces baby bella (cremini) mushrooms, halved
- ¼ cup 0% Greek yogurt
- 2 cloves garlic, thinly sliced
- 1¼ pounds 93% lean ground turkey
- 2 teaspoons spicy brown mustard
- ½ teaspoon fine sea salt
- ¼ teaspoon black pepper
- ¼ cup no-salt-added tomato paste

1. In a food processor, combine the mushrooms, yogurt, and garlic and pulse until the mushrooms are finely chopped.

2. In a large bowl, combine the mushroom mixture, turkey, mustard, salt, and pepper until well mixed. Shape the meat into 4 compact patties about 5 inches across.

3. Preheat the broiler. Broil the burgers 4 inches from the heat, turning over once, until cooked through, about 5 minutes per side.

4. Spread 1 tablespoon tomato paste over each burger and broil for 2 to 3 minutes to glaze.

Per serving: 241 calories • 31g protein • 10g fat (3g saturated) • 1g fiber 35mg calcium • 4mg vitamin C • 7g carbohydrate • 448mg sodium

Chile-Rubbed Pork Tenderloin

Hands-On Time: 10 minutes • **Total Time:** 45 minutes • **Makes:** 4 servings

Rubbing a pork tenderloin with sweet and savory spices lends complex notes to this lean cut of meat. The pork pairs wonderfully with Baked Sweet Potatoes with Peanut Sauce (page 224) or Spicy Braised Collards with Garlic & Raisins (page 215). Leftovers? Place the meat and some shredded reduced-fat pepper jack cheese on one side of a high-fiber wrap (pages 116–117) and fold for a quesadilla, or add some shredded lettuce and salsa to make it a soft taco.

Fat Releasers
Chile powder, cocoa powder, cinnamon, olive oil, pork

2 teaspoons ancho chile powder
1 teaspoon unsweetened cocoa powder
½ teaspoon ground cumin
¼ teaspoon ground cinnamon
¼ teaspoon fine sea salt
1½ tablespoons olive oil
1 pound pork tenderloin

1. In a small bowl, mix together the chile powder, cocoa powder, cumin, cinnamon, salt, and 1 tablespoon of the oil to make a paste. Rub all over the tenderloin and let stand at room temperature for 30 minutes.

2. Preheat the oven to 450°F.

3. In a large ovenproof skillet, heat the remaining oil over medium-high heat until it shimmers. Add the tenderloin and brown on all sides, about 6 minutes.

4. Transfer the skillet to the oven and roast the tenderloin until an instant-read thermometer registers 145°F, about 15 to 20 minutes. Let the meat rest on a cutting board for 10 minutes before slicing.

Per serving: 174 calories • 24g protein • 8g fat (1.5g saturated) • 0.5g fiber 11mg calcium • 1mg vitamin C • 1g carbohydrate • 206mg sodium

Southwestern Chile Verde

Hands-On Time: 25 minutes • **Total Time:** 50 minutes • **Makes:** 4 servings

One serving of the sauce gives you more than 100 percent of your daily requirement for vitamin C (a fat releaser). If you're in the last week of the diet, serve the pork and sauce with whole-wheat couscous (page 227) or brown rice (pages 228–229).

Fat Releasers
Tomatillos, peppers, onion, garlic, pork, olive oil, squash, avocado

¾ **pound tomatillos, halved**

2 **green bell peppers, cut lengthwise into flat panels**

2 **jalapeño peppers**

½ **white onion, quartered lengthwise**

2 **cloves garlic, unpeeled**

½ **cup water**

¼ **teaspoon fine sea salt**

1 **pound pork tenderloin, cut crosswise into 8 slices**

1½ **tablespoons olive oil**

¾ **teaspoon cumin seeds**

¾ **pound zucchini or chayote squash, cut into 1-inch pieces**

1 **avocado, thinly sliced**

1. Preheat the broiler. Broil the tomatillos, bell peppers (skin-side up), jalapeños, onion, and garlic 5 to 6 inches from the heat, turning the onion, garlic, and jalapeños once, until charred and tender, about 15 minutes.

2. Remove the pan from the oven and turn the bell peppers skin-side down. Let the vegetables stand until cool enough to handle. Peel the jalapeño. Peel the garlic and bell peppers. Core the tomatillos.

3. Transfer all of the vegetables to a blender with the water and ⅛ teaspoon of the salt and puree.

4. Pat the pork slices dry and season with the remaining ⅛ teaspoon salt.

5. In a large (12-inch) skillet, heat 1 tablespoon of the oil over medium-high heat. Add the pork and brown it for 2 to 3 minutes on each side. Transfer to a plate.

6. Add the remaining oil to the skillet and cook the cumin seeds until fragrant, 30 seconds. Carefully add the tomatillo puree to the skillet (it will splatter) along with the squash. Cook, stirring frequently, until the squash is crisp-tender and the sauce is reduced by half, about 15 minutes.

7. Return the pork to the pan and simmer, uncovered, until just heated through, about 3 minutes. Spoon onto a platter and top with the avocado slices.

Per serving: 297 calories • 27g protein • 14g fat (2.5g saturated) • 7.5g fiber
49mg calcium • 98mg vitamin C • 18g carbohydrate • 215mg sodium

Grilled Turkey Cutlets with Lemon & Marjoram

Hands-On Time: 15 minutes ● **Total Time:** 45 minutes ● **Makes:** 4 servings

Some supermarkets carry turkey "cutlets" (thick slices of turkey breast) in convenient packages, but others carry only turkey tenderloins. If you can only get the tenderloins, buy two and lightly pound to a ¼-inch thickness. Then cut them in half crosswise to make 4 "cutlets."

Fat Releasers
Garlic, lemon, olive oil, marjoram, black pepper, turkey

- 3 **cloves garlic, minced**
- 2 **tablespoons fresh lemon juice**
- 1½ **tablespoons extra-virgin olive oil**
- 1 **teaspoon dried marjoram**
- ¼ **teaspoon black pepper**
- ⅛ **teaspoon fine sea salt**
- 4 **turkey breast cutlets (4 ounces each)**
- **Lemon wedges, for serving**

1. In a shallow baking dish, whisk together the garlic, lemon juice, oil, marjoram, pepper, and salt. Add the turkey cutlets, turn to coat, and marinate for 30 minutes at room temperature.

2. Preheat a grill or a ridged grill pan to medium-high. Lightly oil the grill grates or grill pan. Grill the turkey, turning once, until just cooked through, about 3 minutes. Serve with the lemon wedges.

Per serving: 172 calories ● 27g protein ● 6g fat (1g saturated) ● 0g fiber
19mg calcium ● 4mg vitamin C ● 1g carbohydrate ● 120mg sodium

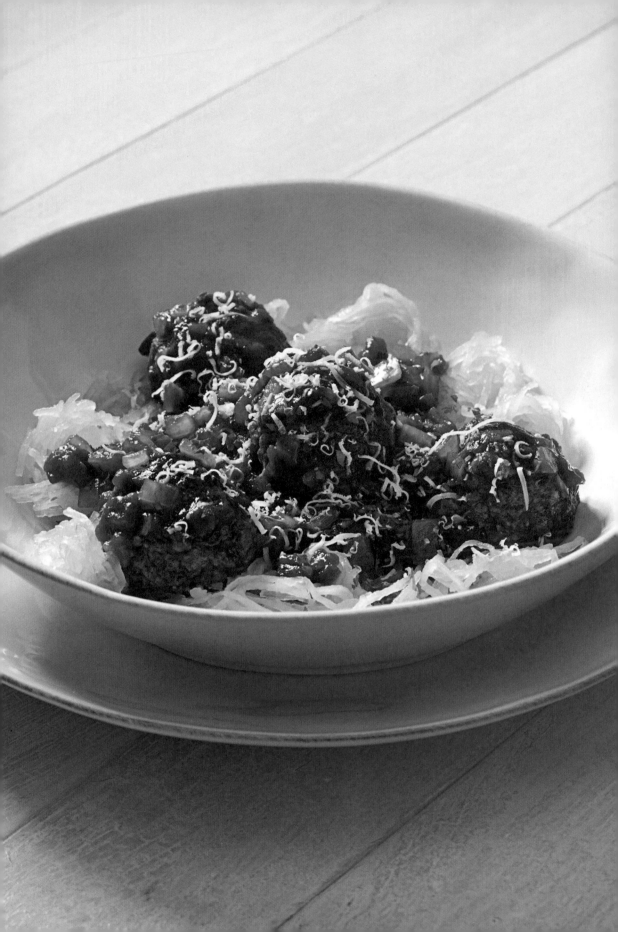

Meatballs & Spaghetti Squash

Hands-On Time: 30 minutes • **Total Time:** 40 minutes • **Makes:** 4 servings

Stretching the meat with fiber-rich oats and using spaghetti squash instead of pasta makes this dish much healthier.

Fat Releasers
Squash, oats, milk, beef, parsley, Parmesan, egg, olive oil, onion, tomatoes, red pepper flakes

- 1 **spaghetti squash (1¾ pounds), halved lengthwise and seeded**
- ¾ **cup quick-cooking oats**
- ½ **cup fat-free milk**
- ¼ **teaspoon fine sea salt**
- ¾ **pound extra-lean (95%) ground beef**
- ½ **cup finely chopped flat-leaf parsley**
- ¼ **cup + 2 tablespoons grated Parmesan cheese**
- 1 **large egg**
- 1 **tablespoon extra-virgin olive oil**
- 1 **onion, chopped**
- 1 **can (14.5 ounces) no-salt-added diced tomatoes**
- ½ **cup water**
- ¼ **teaspoon red pepper flakes**

1. In a large steamer basket set over a pan of simmering water, steam the squash halves, cut-side down, until tender, about 18 minutes. When cool enough to handle, scrape the flesh into strands with a fork. Keep warm.

2. Meanwhile, in a medium bowl, combine the oats, milk, and salt. Let soak for 10 minutes to soften.

3. Add the beef, ¼ cup + 2 tablespoons of the parsley, ¼ cup of the Parmesan, and the egg to the oat mixture. Mix until blended. Form into 16 balls and place on an oiled rimmed baking sheet.

4. Preheat the broiler.

5. In a large skillet, heat the oil over medium heat. Add the onion and cook, stirring occasionally, until softened, 5 to 6 minutes. Add the tomatoes (with juice), water, and pepper flakes and cook, stirring occasionally, until slightly thickened, 5 minutes. Keep warm while you broil the meatballs.

6. Broil the meatballs 5 to 6 inches from heat just until browned and firm, 5 to 6 minutes. Remove from the broiler and add to the tomato sauce and cook, covered, for 5 minutes.

7. Divide the squash among 4 plates and top with 4 meatballs and one-quarter of the sauce. Sprinkle each serving with ½ tablespoon each Parmesan and parsley.

Per serving: 365 calories • 29g protein • 13g fat (4.5g saturated) • 3.5g fiber 222mg calcium • 33mg vitamin C • 33g carbohydrate • 393mg sodium

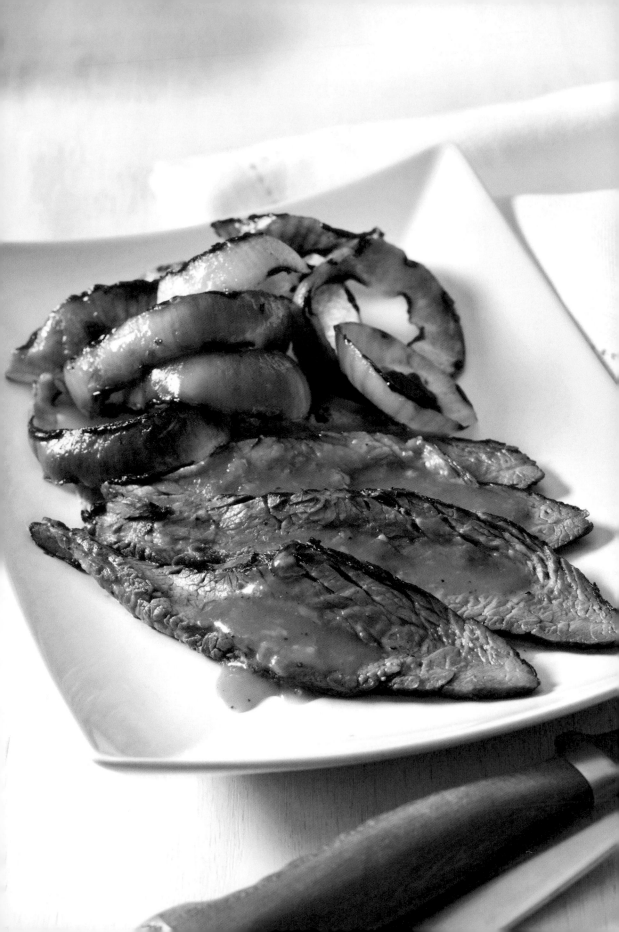

Marinated Flank Steak with Grilled Red Onions

Hands-On Time: 30 minutes • **Total Time:** 1 hour • **Makes:** 4 servings

If you have any leftover steak and onions, chop them well and toss with some baby spinach, field greens, or baby arugula and a little balsamic vinegar for a lunch salad.

Fat Releasers
Orange, ginger, honey, black pepper, beef, onion

- ½ cup fresh orange juice
- 1 teaspoon grated fresh ginger
- 1 teaspoon honey
- ¼ teaspoon fine sea salt
- ¼ teaspoon black pepper
- 1 pound flank steak
- 3 red onions, thickly sliced crosswise

1. In a shallow baking dish, whisk together the orange juice, ginger, honey, salt, and pepper. Add the steak and onions and let marinate for 30 minutes at room temperature. Reserve the marinade.

2. Preheat a grill or a ridged grill pan to medium. Lightly oil the grill grates or grill pan. Grill the onions, turning occasionally, until crisp tender, about 10 minutes. Transfer the onions to a bowl and keep warm.

3. Grill the steak, turning once, until medium-rare, about 10 minutes. Let the meat rest 5 minutes on a cutting board before thinly slicing it across the grain.

4. While the meat is resting, transfer the reserved marinade to a small saucepan and boil until reduced by half, 2 to 3 minutes. Stir in any meat juices accumulated on the cutting board. Serve the meat with the onions and sauce.

Per serving: 256 calories • 26g protein • 8.5g fat (2.5g saturated) • 2.5g fiber 64mg calcium • 24mg vitamin C • 18g carbohydrate • 214mg sodium

Orange Beef with Green Beans, Broccoli & Bok Choy

Hands-On Time: 25 minutes • **Total Time:** 25 minutes • **Makes:** 4 servings

You can swap in other green vegetables if you like: Try Swiss chard instead of bok choy or green bell peppers instead of green beans. If you're in the last phase of the diet, serve the stir-fry with brown rice (pages 228–229) or whole-wheat couscous (page 227).

Fat Releasers
Beef, olive oil, broccoli, ginger, garlic, bok choy, sesame oil

- ¾ **pound flank steak**
- ½ **pound broccoli (1 large or 2 small stalks)**
- 1 **tablespoon cornstarch**
- 1 **tablespoon + 1 teaspoon extra-light olive oil**
- 6 **ounces green beans, halved crosswise**
- 2 **tablespoons chopped fresh ginger**
- 2 **cloves garlic, minced**
- 2 **strips orange zest (2 x ½ inch each)**
- 1 **cup water**
- 1 **bunch bok choy, well washed and cut crosswise into ½-inch-wide ribbons**
- 1 **tablespoon soy sauce**
- 2 **teaspoons toasted (dark) sesame oil**

1. Halve the flank steak lengthwise (in the same direction as the grain of the meat). Then, with your knife at an angle to the cutting board, cut each piece across the grain into thin slices.

2. Separate the broccoli tops from the stems and break into small florets. Peel the stems. If large, halve lengthwise and thinly slice crosswise; if small, just slice crosswise.

3. In a large bowl, toss the beef with the cornstarch until coated.

4. In a large skillet, heat the oil over medium-high heat until hot but not smoking. Add the beef and cook, tossing frequently, until lightly browned, about 3 minutes. Transfer to a bowl.

5. Add the broccoli, green beans, ginger, garlic, and orange zest and cook, tossing frequently, until the vegetables are well coated. Add the water and bok choy and cook until the vegetables are crisp-tender.

6. Return the beef to the pan along with the soy sauce and sesame oil and toss until coated and heated through.

Per serving: 239 calories • 23g protein • 12g fat (3g saturated) • 3.5g fiber 182mg calcium • 108mg vitamin C • 12g carbohydrate • 380mg sodium

Chunky Beef & Vegetable Chili with Red Wine

Hands-On Time: 25 minutes • **Total Time:** 1 hour 40 minutes • **Makes:** 4 servings

Make a double batch of the chili and freeze half for another dinner or for lunches. Divide into 5-cup portions for dinner (to serve four) or 1¼-cup portions for individual lunches. Freeze in small plastic resealable bags and lay the bags flat on a baking sheet until frozen. This will make the chili more compact and easier to stack in the freezer.

Fat Releasers
Olive oil, beef, onion, sweet potato, cocoa, tomatoes, red wine, thyme, zucchini, peas

- 1 tablespoon olive oil
- ¾ pound well-trimmed beef sirloin, cut into ½-inch chunks
- 1 large onion, diced
- 1 sweet potato (10 ounces), peeled and cut into 1-inch chunks
- 1 tablespoon unsweetened cocoa powder
- 2 tablespoons no-salt-added tomato paste
- 1⅓ cups dry red wine
- ½ teaspoon dried thyme
- 1 zucchini (6 ounces), halved lengthwise and cut crosswise into ½-inch-thick half-moons
- 1 cup frozen green peas (no need to thaw)

1. In a Dutch oven, heat the oil over medium heat. Add the beef and cook until browned all over, about 5 minutes. With a slotted spoon, transfer the beef to a plate.

2. Add the onion to the pan and cook, stirring frequently, until tender, about 7 minutes.

3. Stir in the sweet potato and cocoa powder and cook for 1 minute. Add the tomato paste, stirring to coat. Add the wine and thyme and bring to a boil. Return the beef (and any juices from the plate) to the pan, reduce to a simmer, cover, and cook until the sweet potato and meat are tender, about 1 hour 15 minutes.

4. Add the zucchini and cook for 5 minutes. Stir in the peas and cook until heated through, about 2 minutes.

Per 1¼-cup serving: 341 calories • 22g protein • 11g fat (3.5g saturated) • 5g fiber 76mg calcium • 25mg vitamin C • 24g carbohydrate • 100mg sodium

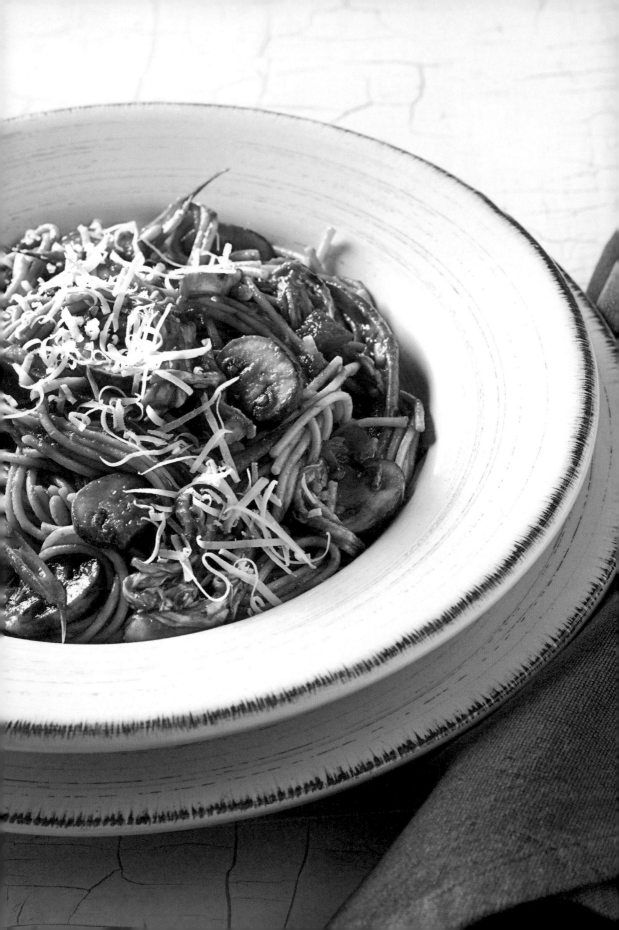

Spaghetti with Super Mushroomy Marinara

Hands-On Time: 10 minutes • **Total Time:** 25 minutes • **Makes:** 4 servings

How do you enjoy spaghetti without all the carbs? Sub in skinny green beans for some of the pasta. You'll have a nice full plate, but you'll be getting a good helping of vegetables at the same time. Look for a brand of bottled marinara with a reasonable amount of sodium (under 450 milligrams per serving if you can find one). Or, ideally, use a homemade marinara where you get to control the amount of salt used.

Fat Releasers
Vinegar, black pepper, mushrooms, tomatoes, turkey, Parmesan cheese

¼ cup water

2 teaspoons red-wine vinegar

¼ teaspoon black pepper

16 ounces sliced baby bella (cremini) mushrooms

2 cups bottled marinara

6 ounces cooked turkey breast, chicken breast, or roast beef, slivered or shredded

6 ounces whole-wheat spaghetti, broken into thirds

1 package (10 ounces) frozen French-cut green beans, thawed

¼ cup shredded Parmesan cheese

1. Bring a large pot of water to a boil for the pasta.

2. In a medium saucepan, combine the ¼ cup water, vinegar, and pepper over medium-high heat. Add the mushrooms, stir to coat, cover, and cook, stirring occasionally, until they are beginning to soften and giving up their liquid, about 5 minutes.

3. Add the marinara and shredded meat and simmer while you cook the pasta.

4. Add the pasta to the boiling water and cook according to package directions.

5. Place the beans in a colander and drain the hot pasta over them. Return both to the pot, add the mushroom sauce, and toss to coat. Sprinkle each serving with 1 tablespoon of the Parmesan.

Per 2-cup serving: 352 calories • 27g protein • 5g fat (1.5g saturated) • 9.5g fiber 157mg calcium • 18mg vitamin C • 53g carbohydrate • 489mg sodium

Baja Fish Tacos with Avocado-Radish Relish & "Crema"

Hands-On Time: 20 minutes • **Total Time:** 25 minutes • **Makes:** 4 servings

This is fun party fare. Put out the fish, relish, "crema," and lettuce in separate bowls and let each person assemble his own taco.

Fat Releasers
Yogurt, chile powder, radishes, avocado, tomatoes, onion, lime, fish, olive oil, lettuce

- ½ cup 0% Greek yogurt
- 1 tablespoon reduced-fat mayonnaise (made with olive oil)
- ½ teaspoon chipotle chile powder
- ½ avocado, diced
- 4 radishes, halved and thinly sliced
- 3 tablespoons finely chopped onion
- 1 tomato, diced
- 2 teaspoons fresh lime juice
- ¾ teaspoon ground coriander
- 2 pinches of fine sea salt
- 1 pound white fish fillets, such as cod, grouper, or snapper
- 2 teaspoons extra-virgin olive oil
- 8 high-fiber whole-wheat tortillas (6 or 7 inches)
- 2 cups shredded lettuce

1. Make the "crema": In a small bowl, stir together the yogurt, mayonnaise, and chile powder. Cover and refrigerate.

2. Make the avocado-radish relish: In a small bowl, stir gently to combine the avocado, radishes, onion, tomato, lime juice, ½ teaspoon of the coriander, and a pinch of the salt. Cover and refrigerate.

3. Preheat the broiler. In a medium bowl, toss the fish with the oil, the remaining ¼ teaspoon coriander, and the remaining pinch of salt. Place the fish on a foil-lined broiler pan and broil 4 inches from the heat until opaque throughout, about 5 minutes.

4. Wrap the tortillas in foil and place in the oven while the broiler is on for 3 to 4 minutes to heat them up (or heat them in the microwave wrapped in paper towels).

5. Top each tortilla with ¼ cup lettuce. Divide the fish among the tortillas and top each with about 1 tablespoon of the relish and a generous tablespoon of the "crema." Serve each person 2 tacos.

Per 2-taco serving: 276 calories • 32g protein • 1g fat (1g saturated) • 17g fiber 143mg calcium • 12mg vitamin C • 27g carbohydrate • 596mg sodium

Balsamic-Glazed Salmon

Hands-On Time: 10 minutes • **Total Time:** 25 minutes • **Makes:** 4 servings

The intense fruitiness and tang of balsamic vinegar marry well with the rich flavor of salmon. As a bonus, vinegar is also a fat releaser. If you have any leftovers, make a lunch salad: baby arugula, chopped tomatoes, a little avocado or asparagus, and some Digest Diet Vinaigrette (page 211) with a little nonfat yogurt stirred in.

Fat Releasers
Vinegar, honey, cayenne pepper, salmon

¼ cup balsamic vinegar

1½ teaspoons honey

⅛ teaspoon fine sea salt

⅛ teaspoon cayenne pepper

4 salmon fillets
(5 ounces each)

1. Preheat the oven to 450°F.
2. In a small saucepan, whisk together the vinegar, honey, salt, and cayenne pepper. Bring to a boil and cook over medium heat until reduced to 2 tablespoons, about 5 minutes. Reserve 1 tablespoon of the balsamic glaze in a small cup.
3. Oil a shallow baking dish and add the salmon. Brush with the remaining 1 tablespoon balsamic glaze. Roast, uncovered, until just cooked through, 10 to 12 minutes.
4. Serve the fish drizzled with the reserved balsamic glaze.

Per serving: 298 calories • 39g protein • 12g fat (2g saturated) • 0g fiber 27mg calcium • 0mg vitamin C • 5g carbohydrate • 161mg sodium

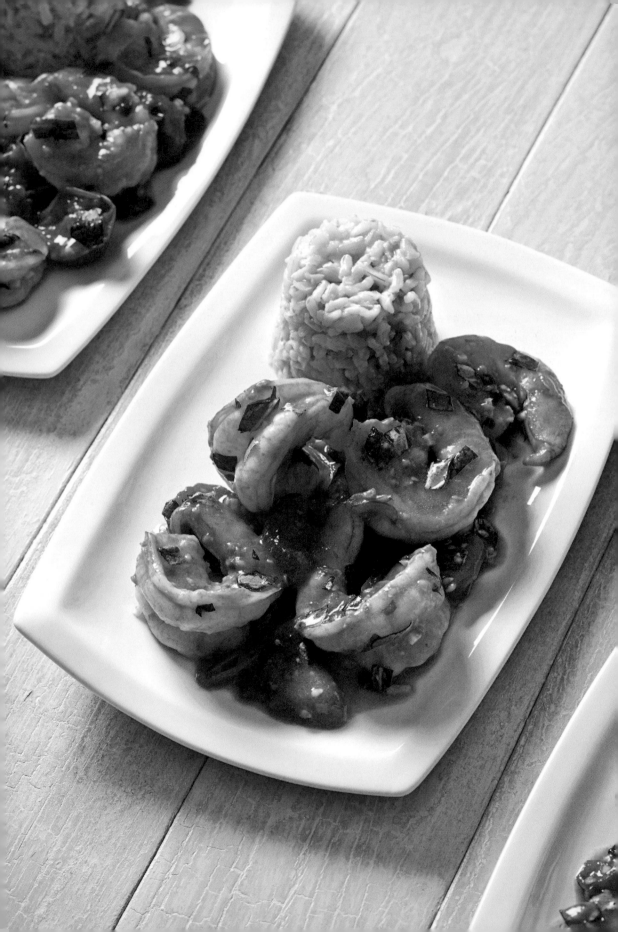

Shrimp Scampi with Cherry Tomatoes & Basil

Hands-On Time: 25 minutes • **Total Time:** 25 minutes • **Makes:** 4 servings

This quick dish of garlic-laced shrimp is a go-to favorite. If you're in the last phase of the diet, serve it with whole-wheat couscous (page 227) or brown rice (pages 228–229). If you use frozen shrimp, look for unpeeled shrimp; the shell helps retain flavor when the shrimp are cooked. Be sure to thaw the shrimp in the refrigerator.

Fat Releasers
Garlic, red pepper flakes, olive oil, tomatoes, shrimp, black pepper, basil

- 2 **cloves garlic, finely chopped**
- ¼ **teaspoon red pepper flakes**
- 1½ **tablespoons extra-virgin olive oil**
- 2 **cups halved cherry tomatoes**
- 1 **pound large shrimp, peeled and deveined**
- ¼ **teaspoon black pepper**
- 3 **tablespoons chopped fresh basil**

1. In a large (12-inch) skillet, cook the garlic and red pepper flakes in the oil over medium heat, stirring occasionally, until pale golden, 1 to 2 minutes.

2. Add the tomatoes and cook, stirring occasionally, until they begin to soften, 3 minutes.

3. Pat the shrimp dry and sprinkle with the black pepper. Add the shrimp to the skillet and cook, turning the shrimp once, until just cooked through, about 4 minutes. Stir in the basil and serve.

Per serving: 143 calories • 16g protein • 6.5g fat (1g saturated) • 1g fiber 76mg calcium • 12mg vitamin C • 5g carbohydrate • 646mg sodium

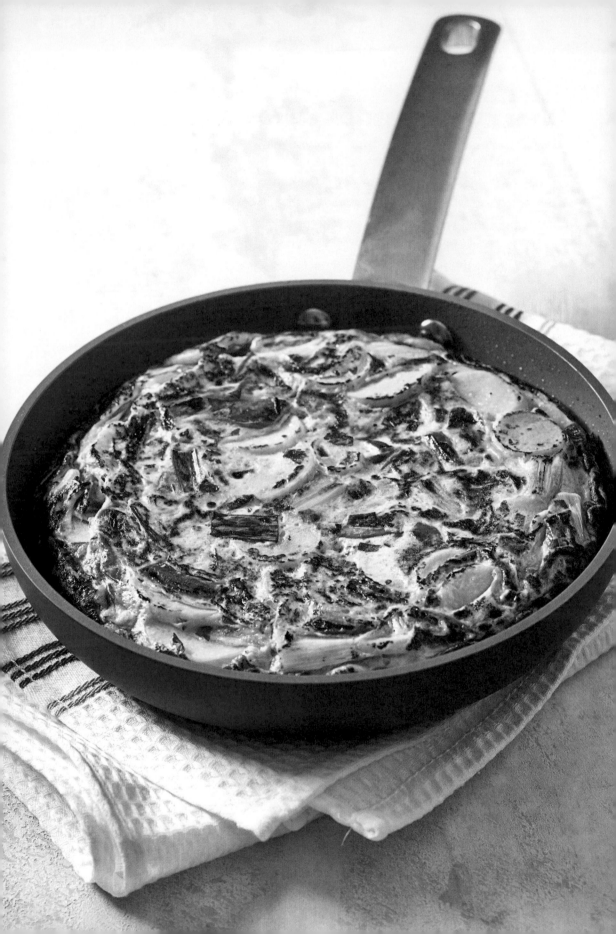

Tri-Color Frittata

Hands-On Time: 25 minutes • **Total Time:** 35 minutes • **Makes:** 4 servings

Frittatas are a good way to get quality protein (eggs) combined with a good helping of vegetables. If you use a variety of colors for the vegetables, you'll be adding not only visual appeal but also a good range of healthful phytochemicals. Leftover frittata makes a spectacular breakfast or lunch: Reheat gently in the microwave or toaster oven, or just have it at room temperature.

Fat Releasers
Tomatoes, olive oil, scallions, squash, egg, Parmesan cheese, parsley, black pepper

- 4 **large plum tomatoes, halved**
- 1½ **tablespoons extra-virgin olive oil**
- 1 **bunch scallions, cut into 1-inch pieces**
- 1 **pound yellow squash, cut into ¼-inch rounds**
- 4 **large eggs**
- 4 **large egg whites**
- 1 **ounce Parmesan cheese, very finely grated**
- 2 **tablespoons chopped flat-leaf parsley**
- ¼ **teaspoon black pepper**
- ⅛ **teaspoon fine sea salt**

1. Preheat the broiler.
2. Scoop out the seeds from the insides of the tomatoes and cut the shells into ¼-inch-thick strips.
3. In a medium (10-inch) ovenproof skillet, heat the oil over medium-high heat until it shimmers. Add the tomatoes, scallions, and squash and cook, stirring frequently, until tender and most of the juices have evaporated, about 10 minutes.
4. In a medium bowl, whisk together the whole eggs and egg whites until blended, then whisk in the Parmesan, parsley, pepper, and salt. Pour the mixture over the vegetables and reduce the heat to medium-low. Cook until the eggs are almost set on top but still runny, about 10 minutes.
5. Transfer the skillet to the oven and broil 5 to 6 inches from the heat just until the top is set and golden, about 2 minutes.

Per serving: 204 calories • 15g protein • 12g fat (3.5g saturated) • 3g fiber 157mg calcium • 36mg vitamin C • 10g carbohydrate • 318mg sodium

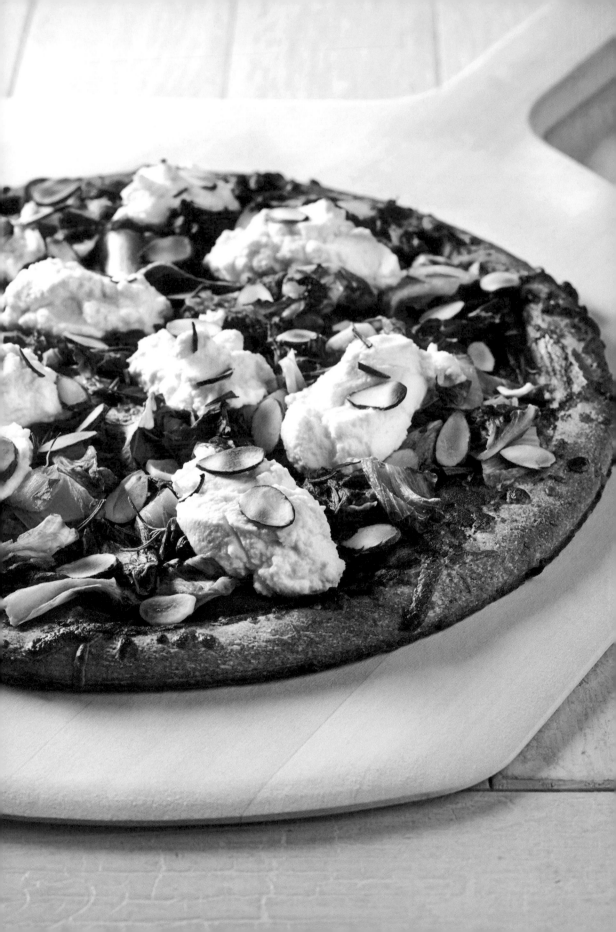

Pizza with Wilted Greens, Ricotta & Almonds

Hands-On Time: 15 minutes • **Total Time:** 30 minutes • **Makes:** 4 servings

Prebaked whole-wheat pizza shells, available in the bread aisle of the supermarket, mean you can have a much healthier pizza on the table in less time than it takes to get delivery. If you prefer, swap in low-fat cottage cheese for the ricotta; to make it super creamy, puree it in the food processor for a minute.

Fat Releasers
Garlic, rosemary, escarole, olive oil, ricotta cheese, black pepper, tomatoes, almonds

- ¼ cup + 2 teaspoons water
- 2 cloves garlic, thinly sliced
- ½ teaspoon chopped fresh or dried rosemary
- 12 ounces escarole, well washed and cut into ½-inch-wide ribbons
- 2 teaspoons extra-virgin olive oil
- 1 thin-crust whole-wheat pizza shell (12-inch)
- 1 cup part-skim ricotta cheese
- ¼ teaspoon fine sea salt
- ¼ teaspoon black pepper
- ¼ cup no-salt-added tomato paste
- 3 tablespoons sliced almonds

1. Preheat the oven to 500°F.

2. In a large (12-inch) skillet, combine ¼ cup of the water, the garlic, and rosemary and bring to a boil.

3. Add the escarole, large handfuls at a time, adding more to the pan as each batch wilts. Cover and cook until the escarole is tender, about 5 minutes. Drain.

4. In a small bowl, whisk together the oil and the remaining 2 teaspoons water. Brush onto the pizza shell and place it on a baking sheet. Bake for 5 minutes.

5. In a small bowl, stir together the ricotta, salt, and pepper.

6. Remove the pizza from the oven and reduce the oven temperature to 375°F. Brush the top of the pizza with the tomato paste. Top with the escarole and then spoonfuls of the ricotta mixture. Sprinkle with the almonds. Bake until the crust is crisp and the almonds start to brown, 3 to 5 minutes. Cut into 8 wedges.

Per 2-wedge serving: 341 calories • 17g protein • 13g fat (5g saturated) • 10g fiber 296mg calcium • 10mg vitamin C • 44g carbohydrate • 603mg sodium

Quinoa Fritters with Spicy Pepper Sauce

Hands-On Time: 20 minutes • **Total Time:** 25 minutes • **Makes:** 4 servings

This protein-rich grain comes in four colors: white, yellow, red, and black. You can make these fritters with any one of the colors of quinoa. They all cook the same way and taste alike, so it's just a matter of appearance. White quinoa is pretty reliably available in supermarkets, but for the other colors, you should check your local natural foods store.

Fat Releasers
Scallions, garlic, quinoa, red pepper, tomatoes, cayenne pepper, egg, Parmesan cheese, feta cheese, olive oil

- 2 **cups water**
- 5 **scallions, halved lengthwise and thinly sliced crosswise**
- 2 **cloves garlic, minced**
- ¼ **teaspoon fine sea salt**
- 1 **cup quinoa, rinsed**
- ½ **cup roasted red pepper**
- 2 **tablespoons no-salt-added tomato paste**
- ⅛ **teaspoon cayenne pepper**
- 4 **large egg whites**
- ½ **cup shredded Parmesan cheese**
- ¼ **cup crumbled reduced-fat feta cheese**
- 2 **tablespoons olive oil**

1. In a medium saucepan, combine the water, scallions, garlic, and salt. Bring to a boil.

2. Add the quinoa and return to a boil. Reduce to a simmer, cover, and cook for 10 minutes. Uncover and cook until the water has evaporated and the quinoa is tender, 2 to 3 minutes longer. Transfer the quinoa mixture to a large bowl and let cool to room temperature.

3. In a food processor, combine the roasted red pepper, tomato paste, and cayenne pepper and process until smooth. Set aside.

4. To the cooled quinoa, add the egg whites, Parmesan, and feta and stir to combine.

5. In a large (12-inch) nonstick skillet, heat 1 tablespoon of the oil over medium heat. Drop four generous ¼ cupfuls of quinoa into the skillet and flatten with a spatula. Cook until golden brown, about 2 minutes per side. Transfer to a plate. Repeat for a total of 8 fritters. Top with the spicy pepper sauce.

Per 2-fritter serving: 312 calories • 16g protein • 13g fat (3.5g saturated) • 4g fiber 192mg calcium • 15mg vitamin C • 32g carbohydrate • 455mg sodium

Japanese Spinach Salad with Carrot-Sesame Dressing

Hands-On Time: 10 minutes • **Total Time:** 15 minutes • **Makes:** 4 servings

Make a double batch of dressing and store it in the fridge, where it'll keep for a week. Try spooning some over steamed vegetables or as a sauce for cooked chicken.

Fat Releasers
Ginger, vinegar, honey, sesame oil, olive oil, spinach

- 1 **large carrot, thinly sliced (generous ¾ cup)**
- 1 **tablespoon chopped fresh ginger**
- 1 **tablespoon rice vinegar or apple-cider vinegar**
- 1 **teaspoon honey**
- 1 **teaspoon toasted (dark) sesame oil**
- 1 **teaspoon extra-light olive oil**
- ⅛ **teaspoon fine sea salt**
- 1 **bag (5 ounces) baby spinach**

1. In a small saucepan, combine the carrot, ginger, and enough water to cover by 2 inches. Bring to a boil over high heat. Reduce to a simmer, cover, and cook until the carrot is very tender, about 7 minutes.

2. Transfer the carrot and 2 tablespoons of the cooking liquid to a mini chopper and puree until smooth. Add the vinegar, honey, sesame oil, olive oil, and salt. Puree until well combined and a thin consistency. If not using right away, store in the fridge.

3. Place the spinach in a large bowl, add the dressing, and toss to coat.

Per serving: 53 calories • 1g protein • 2.5g fat (0.5g saturated) • 2.5g fiber 35mg calcium • 7mg vitamin C • 8g carbohydrate • 149mg sodium

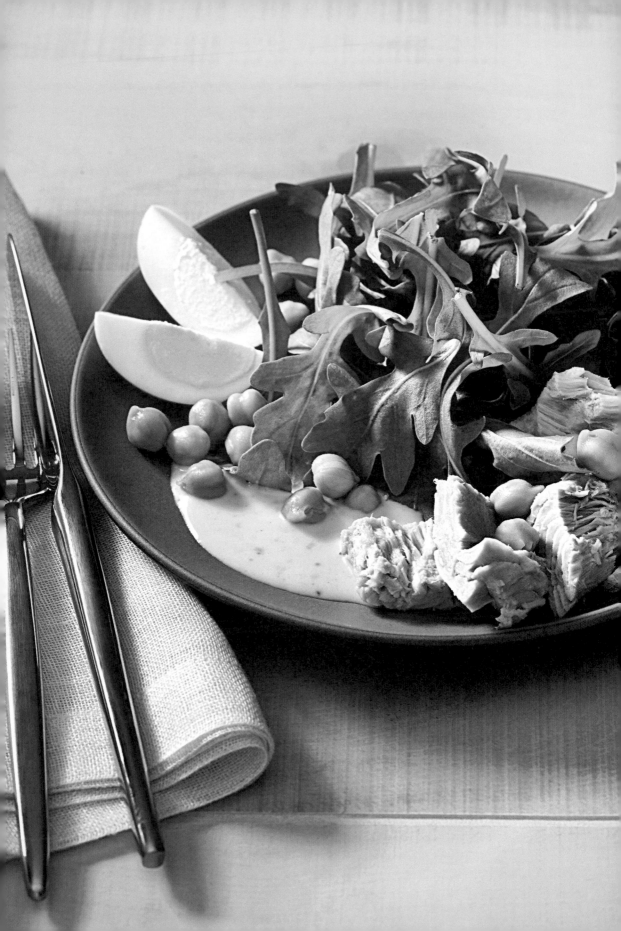

Tuna, Egg & Chickpea Salad with Buttermilk Dressing

Hands-On Time: 5 minutes • **Total Time:** 20 minutes • **Makes:** 4 servings

While you're preparing this dish, cook a half-dozen or so hard-boiled eggs; peel only what you need for the salad and refrigerate the remainder. Hard-boiled eggs are great to have on hand for a quick high-protein snack.

Fat Releasers
Egg, buttermilk, oregano, black pepper, chickpeas, arugula, tuna

2 large eggs

½ cup low-fat buttermilk

2 tablespoons reduced-fat mayonnaise (made with olive oil)

¼ teaspoon dried oregano

⅛ teaspoon fine sea salt

⅛ teaspoon black pepper

1 can (15 ounces) low-sodium chickpeas, rinsed and drained

1 package (5 ounces) baby arugula

2 cans (5 ounces each) water-packed albacore tuna, drained

1. Place the eggs in a small saucepan with cold water to cover by 2 inches. Bring to a boil. Remove from the heat, cover, and let stand 12 minutes. Run the eggs under cold water until cool, then peel the eggs and cut them into quarters. Set aside.

2. In a large bowl, whisk together the buttermilk, mayo, oregano, salt, and pepper. Add the chickpeas and arugula. Toss to combine.

3. Divide the chickpea mixture among 4 plates. Top with the tuna and eggs.

Per serving: 282 calories • 28g protein • 8g fat (1.5g saturated) • 5g fiber
144mg calcium • 4mg vitamin C • 24g carbohydrate • 495mg sodium

Kale Salad with Feta, Grapes & Pumpkin Seeds

Hands-On Time: 20 minutes • **Total Time:** 20 minutes • **Makes:** 4 servings

Kale is a hearty but mild-flavored green that works really well paired with feta and sweet red grapes. And you can easily throw in a little extra protein if you like: Two to three ounces of chopped cooked chicken, turkey, or shrimp will work. Because the greens are sturdy, this salad is perfect to pack for a workday lunch.

Fat Releasers
Kale, pumpkin seeds, olive oil, vinegar, red grapes, feta cheese

- ¾ **pound kale, tough ribs removed and leaves cut crosswise into 2-inch pieces (9 cups)**
- ¼ **cup hulled pumpkin seeds**
- 1½ **tablespoons extra-virgin olive oil**
- 1½ **tablespoons red-wine vinegar**
- 1½ **cups halved seedless red grapes**
- 5 **ounces crumbled reduced-fat feta cheese**

1. In a large steamer basket or colander set over a pan of simmering water, steam the kale until tender, 3 to 5 minutes. Rinse under cold water to stop the cooking. Pat dry.

2. In a small skillet, cook the pumpkin seeds over low heat until the seeds begin to pop and are fragrant, about 3 minutes. Scrape them out of the pan to stop further cooking and set aside.

3. In a large bowl, whisk together the oil and vinegar. Add the kale, grapes, and feta and toss gently to combine.

4. Top each serving with 1 tablespoon of the pumpkin seeds.

Per 2-cup serving: 228 calories • 12g protein • 14g fat (4.5g saturated) • 3.5g fiber 178mg calcium • 43mg vitamin C • 17g carbohydrate • 512mg sodium

Avocado, Orange & Romaine Salad with Pumpkin Seeds

Hands-On Time: 15 minutes • **Total Time:** 15 minutes • **Makes:** 4 servings

This refreshing salad goes well with any meal, especially the Hearty Mexican Chicken Soup (page 169), and it is perfect for the winter when oranges are at their best. Turn the salad into a main dish by adding 1½ cups shredded grilled chicken and sprinkling with 1 ounce crumbled reduced-fat goat or feta cheese.

Fat Releasers
Lettuce, orange, avocado, honey, cinnamon, black pepper, cayenne pepper, pumpkin seeds

- 4 **cups torn romaine lettuce**
- 2 **seedless oranges, peeled and sliced**
- 1 **avocado, sliced**
- 2 **tablespoons fresh orange juice**
- 1 **teaspoon honey**
- ¼ **teaspoon ground cinnamon**
- ⅛ **teaspoon fine sea salt**
- ⅛ **teaspoon black pepper**
  Pinch of cayenne pepper
- 2 **tablespoons hulled toasted pumpkin seeds**

1. Put the lettuce on a platter and arrange the orange and the avocado slices on top.

2. In a small bowl, whisk together the orange juice, honey, cinnamon, salt, black pepper, and cayenne pepper. Drizzle over the salad and sprinkle with the pumpkin seeds.

Per serving: 131 calories • 3g protein • 7.5g fat (1g saturated) • 5g fiber 55mg calcium • 50mg vitamin C • 16g carbohydrate • 80mg sodium

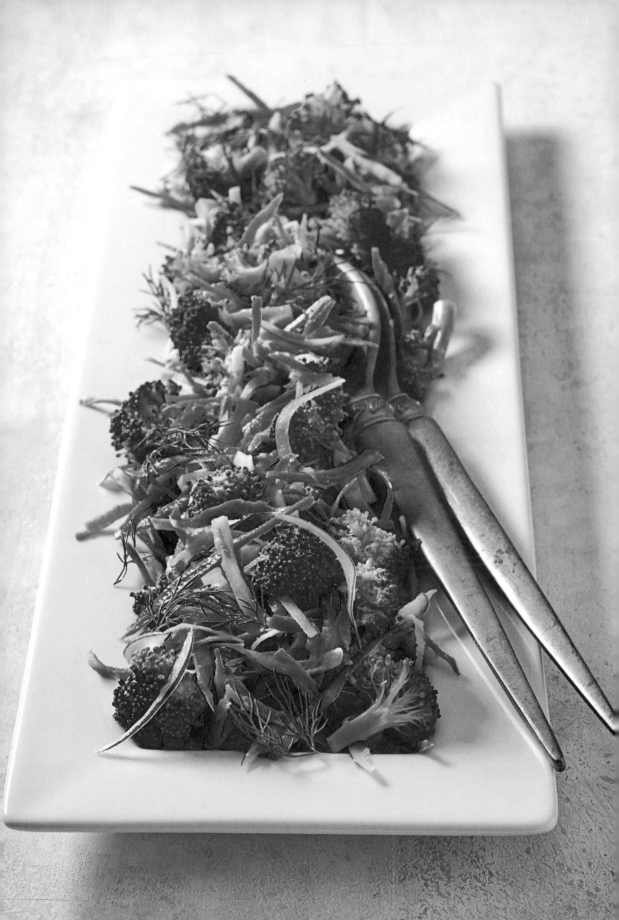

Tangy Broccoli Slaw

Hands-On Time: 10 minutes • **Total Time:** 50 minutes • **Makes:** 4 servings

Some markets may carry packaged broccoli slaw, but the vitamin C in the broccoli begins to diminish once the vegetable has been cut, and it loses even more as it sits exposed to the light in the produce section. You're much better off starting with fresh. But in a pinch, it would be better to use precut broccoli than to not make this at all: You'll need about 4 cups.

Fat Releasers
Broccoli, onion, buttermilk, vinegar, black pepper

1 **pound broccoli**

1 **large carrot, coarsely grated**

¼ **cup finely chopped red onion**

3 **tablespoons chopped fresh dill**

¾ **cup low-fat buttermilk**

1 **tablespoon vinegar (preferably malt)**

¼ **teaspoon fine sea salt**

¼ **teaspoon black pepper**

1. Separate the broccoli florets and stems. Cut the florets into ½-inch pieces. Peel the stem and coarsely grate. Toss with the carrot and onion in a large bowl.

2. In a small bowl, combine the dill, buttermilk, vinegar, salt, and pepper. Add to the vegetables and toss. Let stand 30 minutes, stirring occasionally, to allow flavors to blend.

Per 1¼-cup serving: 69 calories • 5g protein • 1g fat (0.5g saturated) • 3.5g fiber 116mg calcium • 104mg vitamin C • 12g carbohydrate • 244mg sodium

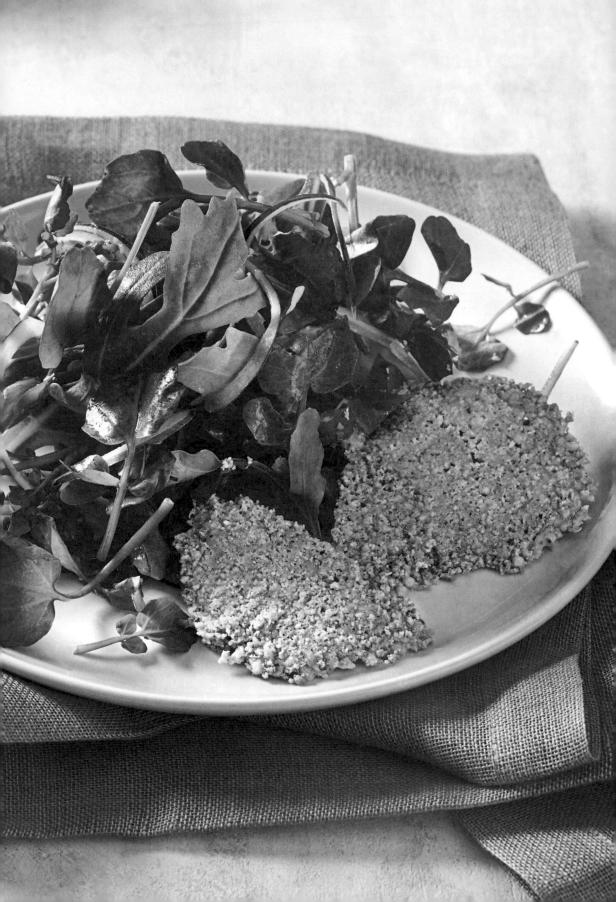

Watercress-Arugula Salad with Parmesan "Crackers"

Hands-On Time: 15 minutes • **Total Time:** 15 minutes • **Makes:** 4 servings

You're getting a major cruciferous vegetable hit from the watercress and arugula—not to mention from the mustard in the dressing. But this also means that this is a fairly pungent salad. If you prefer, you can lighten the pungency by swapping in shredded romaine lettuce for some of the watercress or arugula.

Fat Releasers
Watercress, arugula, onion, olive oil, lemon, Parmesan cheese, almonds, black pepper

- 1 **bunch watercress (6 ounces), tough stems trimmed, coarsely chopped**
- 4 **cups packed baby arugula (about 4 ounces)**
- ½ **small red onion, very thinly slivered**
- 3 **tablespoons Digest Diet Vinaigrette (page 211) made with lemon juice and no herbs**
- 8 **Parmesan "Crackers" (page 210)**

1. In a large salad bowl, toss together the watercress, arugula, and onion.

2. Add the vinaigrette and toss again to coat. Serve each salad with 2 Parmesan "crackers."

Per serving: 70 calories • 3g protein • 5g fat (1g saturated) • 1.5g fiber 122mg calcium • 26mg vitamin C • 5g carbohydrate • 92mg sodium

Parmesan "Crackers"

Hands-On Time: 5 minutes • **Total Time:** 15 minutes • **Makes:** 8 crackers

Experiment with these super-easy garnishes. Try ground-up pistachios or walnuts instead of almond meal.

Fat Releasers
Parmesan cheese, almonds, black pepper

¼ cup + 2 tablespoons grated
   Parmesan cheese
 2 tablespoons almond meal
¼ teaspoon black pepper

1. Preheat the oven to 375°F. Line a baking sheet with parchment paper or a nonstick liner.

2. In a small bowl, combine the Parmesan, almond meal, and pepper. Spoon 1-tablespoon mounds of the mixture onto the baking sheet, 4 inches apart. With the back of the measuring spoon, gently press each into a round about 2½ inches across (make sure there are no gaps in the mixture).

3. Bake until turning golden all over, about 10 minutes. Let cool for 3 minutes on the baking sheet, then carefully transfer (they're fragile) to a wire rack to cool.

Per cracker: 26 calories • 2g protein • 2g fat (1g saturated) • 0g fiber • 45mg calcium 0mg vitamin C • 0g carbohydrate • 58mg sodium

Digest Diet Vinaigrette

Hands-On Time: 5 minutes • **Total Time:** 5 minutes • **Makes:** 1 cup

To avoid overdressing a salad, always toss the greens with the dressing before serving so you can get even coverage and control how much gets used. And only toss what you'll eat that day; dressed salads don't store well.

Fat Releasers
Garlic, lemon/lime or vinegar, black pepper, olive oil

1 clove garlic
½ cup fresh lemon juice, fresh lime juice, or vinegar (red-wine, white-wine, sherry, rice, red balsamic, white balsamic)
2 tablespoons Dijon mustard
½ teaspoon dried tarragon, oregano, mint, or dill (optional)
½ teaspoon black pepper
¼ cup + 1 tablespoon extra-virgin olive oil

1. Grate the garlic on a citrus zester into a small screw-top jar or any tight-sealing container. Add the juice or vinegar, mustard, herb (if using), and pepper. Shake well to combine.

2. Add the oil and shake to emulsify. If you have the time, let the dressing sit for a while so the garlic can flavor the oil. Store in the refrigerator.

Per tablespoon: 41 calories • 0g protein • 4g fat (0.5g saturated) • 0g fiber 1mg calcium • 3mg vitamin C • 1g carbohydrate • 45mg sodium

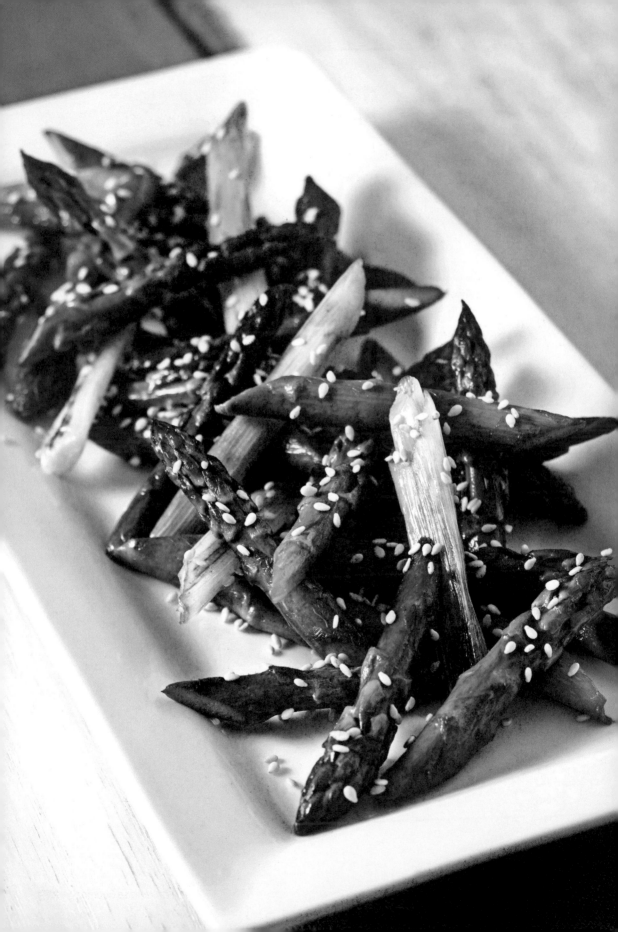

Stir-Fried Asparagus & Scallions

Hands-On Time: 15 minutes • **Total Time:** 15 minutes • **Makes:** 4 servings

Choose slender asparagus, but not the super-skinny ones, for this dish. Save any leftovers for a lunch salad: Toss the asparagus with some whole-wheat couscous (page 227), black beans (page 222), reduced-fat goat cheese or feta cheese, lemon juice, and black pepper.

Fat Releasers
Olive oil, scallions, asparagus, sesame seeds

1 tablespoon extra-virgin olive oil

⅛ teaspoon coarse sea salt

1 bunch scallions, cut into 2-inch lengths

1 bunch asparagus, cut into 2-inch lengths

1 tablespoon toasted sesame seeds

1. Heat the oil and salt in a wok or large skillet over medium-high heat until hot but not smoking. Add the scallions and stir-fry for 2 minutes.

2. Add the asparagus and stir-fry just until crisp-tender, 4 to 5 minutes. Serve sprinkled with the sesame seeds.

Per ½-cup serving: 67 calories • 2g protein • 5g fat (0.5g saturated) • 2g fiber 36mg calcium • 10mg vitamin C • 5g carbohydrate • 74mg sodium

Olive Oil–Roasted Brussels Sprouts

Hands-On Time: 5 minutes • **Total Time:** 20 minutes • **Makes:** 4 servings

You can easily scale up this simple recipe, especially if you want to make extras for snacks. Or use leftovers to make a salad: Toss them with salad greens, some toasted walnuts, and Digest Diet Vinaigrette (page 211) made with lemon juice. Make the salad a main course by adding some shredded cooked turkey, chicken, or shrimp.

Fat Releasers
Brussels sprouts, olive oil, black pepper

¾ **pound Brussels sprouts, halved**

1½ **tablespoons olive oil**

¼ **teaspoon black pepper**

⅛ **teaspoon fine sea salt**

1. Preheat the oven to 425°F.

2. Toss all the ingredients together on a rimmed baking sheet and roast, stirring occasionally, until the sprouts are golden and crisp-tender, about 15 minutes.

Per 1-cup serving: 78 calories • 3g protein • 5.5g fat (1g saturated) • 3g fiber 33mg calcium • 65mg vitamin C • 7g carbohydrate • 92mg sodium

Spicy Braised Collards with Garlic & Raisins

Hands-On Time: 20 minutes • **Total Time:** 30 minutes • **Makes:** 4 servings

Though by regional tradition in this country, collards are often stewed to within an inch of their life, they don't actually need a lot of cooking to turn out tender and mild.

Fat Releasers
Olive oil, garlic, red pepper flakes, collard greens

¼ cup raisins
¼ cup hot water
1 tablespoon olive oil
2 cloves garlic, thinly sliced
¼ teaspoon red pepper flakes
1 pound collard greens, thick stems removed, well washed and cut crosswise into wide ribbons
¼ teaspoon fine sea salt

1. In a small bowl, add the raisins to the water and let stand for 10 minutes to plump.

2. Meanwhile, in a large (12-inch) skillet, heat the oil over medium-low heat. Add the garlic and pepper flakes. Cook, stirring occasionally, until the garlic is tender, about 3 minutes.

3. Add the collards, salt, raisins (with the soaking liquid) and cook, stirring occasionally, until the collards are tender, about 10 minutes.

Per ¾-cup serving: 98 calories • 3g protein • 4g fat (0.5g saturated) • 4g fiber 192mg calcium • 25mg vitamin C • 15g carbohydrate • 168mg sodium

Green Peas & Sautéed Shallots with Thai Herbs

Hands-On Time: 15 minutes • **Total Time:** 15 minutes • **Makes:** 4 servings

Peas may pack a few more calories than other "green" vegetables, but they also pack an impressive amount of soluble fiber and the B vitamin folate. For a quick snack, stir leftover peas into fat-free cottage cheese.

Fat Releasers
Olive oil, peas, basil, lime

2 teaspoons extra-virgin olive oil

Pinch of fine sea salt

¼ cup water

3 large shallots or 1 small red onion, very thinly sliced

1 package (10 ounces) frozen green peas, thawed

2 tablespoons chopped fresh mint

2 tablespoons chopped fresh basil

½ lime, zested and juiced

1. In a large (12-inch) nonstick skillet, stir together the oil, salt, and water. Add the shallots and stir to coat. Bring to a simmer over medium-high heat, cover, and cook until softened and the water is nearly evaporated, about 3 minutes.

2. Uncover, reduce the heat to medium, and cook, stirring occasionally, until the shallots are beginning to brown, about 5 minutes. (If at any point the pan is getting too dry, add a splash of water and keep going.)

3. Stir in the peas, mint, basil, lime zest, and lime juice and cook to heat through, about 1 minute.

Per ⅔-cup serving: 118 calories • 5g protein • 2.5g fat (0.5g saturated) • 3.5g fiber 46mg calcium • 19mg vitamin C • 20g carbohydrate • 119mg sodium

Almond-Parmesan Cauliflower au Gratin

Hands-On Time: 5 minutes • **Total Time:** 25 minutes • **Makes:** 4 servings

The leftovers from this make a great snack. You might even want to roast extra just so you can have these on hand. Just double all the ingredients and roast in a 9 x 13-inch pan.

Fat Releasers
Cauliflower, almonds, Parmesan cheese, lemon

- 1 bag (16 ounces) frozen cauliflower florets, thawed
- Freshly ground black pepper
- Generous pinch of fine sea salt
- 2 tablespoons almond meal or flaxseed meal
- 2 tablespoons grated Parmesan cheese
- ¼ teaspoon paprika (smoked, hot, or sweet)
- Lemon wedges, for serving (optional)

1. Preheat the oven to 400°F. Lightly spray a 7 x 11-inch baking dish with olive oil.

2. Arrange the cauliflower in the baking dish in a single layer. Spray very lightly with olive oil. Sprinkle with a few good grinds of black pepper and a generous pinch of salt. Roast for 10 minutes (to heat up the cauliflower).

3. Meanwhile, in a small bowl, stir together the almond or flaxseed meal, Parmesan, and paprika.

4. Remove the cauliflower from the oven and sprinkle with the Parmesan mixture. Return to the oven and bake until lightly browned on the top, 10 to 12 minutes.

5. Serve with lemon wedges for squeezing over the cauliflower, if desired.

Per ½-cup serving: 69 calories • 4g protein • 4g fat (0.5g saturated) • 3g fiber 62mg calcium • 55mg vitamin C • 6g carbohydrate • 100mg sodium

Edamame Mash with Parmesan

Hands-On Time: 5 minutes • **Total Time:** 20 minutes • **Makes:** 4 servings

This is good as a side dish or as a dip for vegetables. Or you can even thin the edamame mash with broth and toss with strands of spaghetti squash for a bowl of super healthy "pasta."

Fat Releasers
Edamame, garlic, olive oil, lemon, Parmesan cheese

1½ cups frozen shelled edamame

2 cloves garlic, thinly sliced

2 teaspoons olive oil

½ teaspoon grated lemon zest

1 tablespoon fresh lemon juice

¼ teaspoon fine sea salt

¼ cup grated Parmesan cheese

1. In a pot of boiling water, cook the edamame and garlic until tender, about 5 minutes. Measure out ½ cup of the cooking liquid and reserve. Drain the edamame and garlic and transfer to a food processor.

2. Add the ½ cup reserved cooking liquid, the oil, lemon zest, lemon juice, and salt to the processor and puree until smooth. Add the Parmesan and pulse until combined. Serve hot.

Per generous ⅓-cup serving: 120 calories • 10g protein • 6.5g fat (1g saturated) 3g fiber • 89mg calcium • 2mg vitamin C • 6g carbohydrate • 226mg sodium

Peperonata with Fennel

Hands-On Time: 15 minutes • **Total Time:** 35 minutes • **Makes:** 4 servings

Serve these Italian-style peppers as a hot side dish or as a meatless main dish over brown rice (pages 228–229) or whole-wheat couscous (page 227). It's also delicious cold. Pack some for lunch and top it with 1 to 2 tablespoons of fat-free ricotta cheese. If your market carries presliced bell peppers, save yourself some prep time and use them (even if you sacrifice some vitamin C content). Don't worry about what color they are, but try to have at least one that isn't green.

Fat Releasers
Olive oil, garlic, black pepper, bell peppers, tomatoes

---

1 **tablespoon extra-virgin olive oil**

2 **cloves garlic, minced**

¼ **teaspoon black pepper**
   Generous pinch of fine sea salt

½ **cup water**

1 **small fennel bulb, cut into short ½-inch-wide strips**

3 **large bell peppers, seeded and cut into short ½-inch-wide strips**

1 **can (14.5 ounces) no-salt-added diced tomatoes**

1. In a Dutch oven, combine the oil, garlic, black pepper, salt, and ¼ cup of the water. Bring to a boil over medium-high heat.

2. Add the fennel and stir to coat. Cover and cook, stirring once or twice, until the water evaporates and the fennel is beginning to soften, about 5 minutes.

3. Stir in the bell peppers and the remaining ¼ cup water. Cover and cook, stirring once or twice, until the peppers are beginning to soften, about 5 minutes.

4. Add the tomatoes and reduce the heat to medium-low. Cover and cook until the vegetables are soft, about 20 minutes. Check periodically to be sure there is still some liquid in the pan, adding a dash of water if it looks like it's in danger of sticking.

Per 1½-cup serving: 108 calories • 3g protein • 4g fat (0.5g saturated) • 4.5g fiber 60mg calcium • 195mg vitamin C • 17g carbohydrate • 87mg sodium

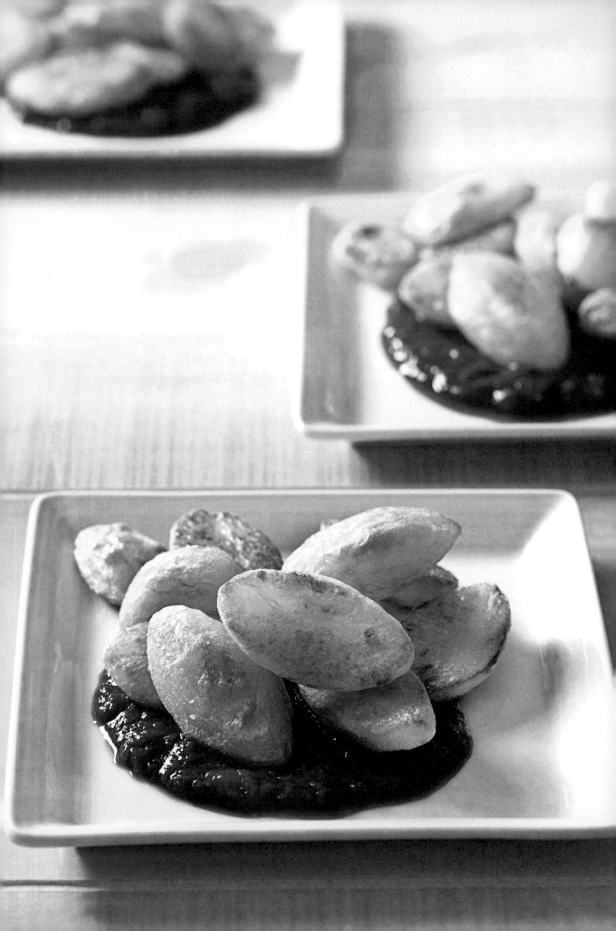

Potatoes with Spicy Paprika-Pepper Sauce

Hands-On Time: 10 minutes • **Total Time:** 35 minutes • **Makes:** 4 servings

If you like, you can prep for this dish the day before. Boil, peel, and cut up the potatoes and store in the fridge. Make the pepper sauce and refrigerate separately. When you're ready to make dinner, all you have to do is sauté the potatoes. You can reheat the sauce or serve it at room temperature.

Fat Releasers
Red pepper, tomatoes, cayenne pepper, olive oil

1 **pound boiling potatoes**
½ **cup roasted red peppers**
2 **teaspoons no-salt-added tomato paste**
1 **teaspoon paprika**
¼ **teaspoon fine sea salt**
⅛ **teaspoon cayenne pepper**
1 **tablespoon + 1 teaspoon extra-virgin olive oil**

1. In a pot of boiling water, cook the potatoes until tender, about 20 minutes. Drain. When cool enough to handle, peel and cut the potatoes into ½-inch chunks.

2. Meanwhile, in a blender, combine the roasted peppers, tomato paste, paprika, salt, and cayenne pepper. Puree until smooth.

3. In a large (12-inch) nonstick skillet, heat the oil over medium heat. Add the potatoes and cook, tossing frequently, until lightly crisped, about 5 minutes.

4. Serve the potatoes with the pepper sauce, or toss the potatoes with the sauce before serving, if desired.

Per serving: 128 calories • 2g protein • 5g fat (0.5g saturated) • 2.5g fiber 4mg calcium • 20mg vitamin C • 20g carbohydrate • 195mg sodium

Beautiful Big-Batch Beans

Hands-On Time: 5 minutes • **Total Time:** 1 hour + soaking time • **Makes:** 6 cups

You can use this method and the seasonings for any type of bean. We chose black beans because they are very flavorful and have the highest level of antioxidant activity of all the beans. Keep in mind that bigger beans (like kidney beans) will take longer to cook.

Fat Releaser
Beans

1 **pound dried black beans**
1½ **teaspoons coarse sea salt**
SEASONING (opposite)

1. Soak the beans overnight in enough water to cover by 2 inches. Or quick-soak: Combine the beans and water and bring to a rolling boil. Turn off the heat, cover, and let the beans soak for 1 hour.

2. Rinse and drain the soaked beans and place in a large saucepan with fresh water to cover by 1 to 2 inches. Add the salt and SEASONING. Bring to a boil over medium-high heat, reduce to a high simmer, partially cover, and cook until the beans are tender, 45 minutes to 1 hour. Keep an eye on the liquid level to make sure the beans are always just barely covered with water.

3. Reserving the cooking liquid, drain the beans. Scoop ½-cup portions into small freezer containers. If you want to keep the flavorful liquid, divide it evenly among the containers once you have filled them with beans. Freeze the beans until ready to use.

Per ½-cup serving: 119 calories • 8g protein • 0.5g fat (0g saturated) • 8g fiber 24mg calcium • 0mg vitamin C • 21g carbohydrate • 240mg sodium

▶ SEASONINGS

Italianesque: 1 small diced red onion, 4 minced garlic cloves, and 1 tablespoon Italian herb seasoning
Fat Releasers: Onion, garlic
Per ½-cup serving: 125 calories • 8g protein • 0.5g fat (0g saturated) • 8g fiber
27mg calcium • 1mg vitamin C • 22g carbohydrate • 257mg sodium

Three-Pepper: 1 diced green bell pepper, 1 seeded and minced serrano or small jalapeño pepper, and 1 teaspoon black pepper
Fat Releasers: Bell pepper, chile pepper, black pepper
Per ½-cup serving: 121 calories • 8g protein • 0.5g fat (0g saturated) • 8g fiber
26mg calcium • 8mg vitamin C • 22g carbohydrate • 241mg sodium

Thai: 4 chopped scallions, 3 minced garlic cloves, 1 tablespoon dried mint, 2 teaspoons dried basil, and grated zest of 1 lime (optional)
Fat Releasers: Scallions, garlic, basil
Per ½-cup serving: 122 calories • 8g protein • 0.5g fat (0g saturated) • 8g fiber
34mg calcium • 1mg vitamin C • 22g carbohydrate • 242mg sodium

Barbecue: 3 minced garlic cloves and 1 tablespoon smoked paprika. After the beans are cooked, stir in 1 can (14.5 ounces) no-salt-added diced tomatoes (with juice) and simmer, uncovered, for another 15 minutes.
Fat Releasers: Garlic, tomatoes
Per ½-cup serving: 129 calories • 8g protein • 0.5g fat (0g saturated) • 8g fiber
32mg calcium • 6mg vitamin C • 23g carbohydrate • 245mg sodium

Baked Sweet Potatoes with Peanut Sauce

Hands-On Time: 20 minutes • **Total Time:** 50 minutes • **Makes:** 6 servings

Once you taste these Asian-flavored sweet potatoes, you will forget all about using marshmallows! This dish hits all the right spicy notes and could even grace a Thanksgiving meal. If there are leftovers, mash the potatoes and add some low-sodium chicken broth and fresh lime juice for a great lunch soup.

Fat Releasers
Sweet potatoes, orange, olive oil, honey, peanut butter, ginger, scallions

1½ **pounds sweet potatoes, peeled and cut crosswise into 1-inch-thick slices**

¼ **cup fresh orange juice**

1½ **teaspoons olive oil**

1 **teaspoon honey**

¼ **teaspoon fine sea salt**

1½ **tablespoons natural peanut butter**

1 **teaspoon grated fresh ginger**

1 **scallion, finely chopped**

3–4 **tablespoons hot water**

1 **tablespoon chopped fresh cilantro**

1. Preheat the oven to 400°F.

2. Arrange the sweet potatoes, slightly overlapping, in a 7- x 11-inch baking dish.

3. In a small bowl, mix together the orange juice, oil, honey, and ⅛ teaspoon of the salt. Drizzle the mixture over the sweet potatoes, cover the dish with foil, and bake until the sweet potatoes are tender, about 30 minutes.

4. Meanwhile, in a small bowl, stir together the peanut butter, ginger, half of the scallions, the remaining ⅛ teaspoon salt, and the hot water until blended.

5. Serve the sweet potatoes drizzled with the peanut sauce and sprinkled with the cilantro and remaining scallions.

Per serving: 167 calories • 3g protein • 5g fat (0.5g saturated) • 4g fiber 40mg calcium • 24mg vitamin C • 28g carbohydrate • 182mg sodium

Orange-Chipotle Broccoli Rabe

Hands-On Time: 10 minutes • **Total Time:** 20 minutes • **Makes:** 4 servings

The bitterness in broccoli rabe comes from healthful anticancer compounds, but if you're not a fan of bitter vegetables, make this with mild broccolini (also called broccolette) instead. It'll still be very good for you. Leftovers make a good lunch salad: Toss with a little balsamic vinegar and some tuna, shredded cooked chicken, or chickpeas.

Fat Releasers
Broccoli rabe,
olive oil, garlic,
orange,
chile powder

- 1 **bunch (1¼ pounds) broccoli rabe or broccolini**
- 1 **tablespoon extra-virgin olive oil**
- 3 **cloves garlic, chopped**
- ½ **orange, zested and juiced**
- ¼ **cup water**
- ¼ **teaspoon chipotle chile powder**
- ⅛ **teaspoon fine sea salt**

1. Trim off the tough stem ends from the broccoli rabe (or broccolini) and cut crosswise into 1-inch pieces.

2. In a large (12-inch) nonstick skillet, combine the oil, garlic, and orange juice. Cook over medium heat until the garlic is fragrant and softened, about 2 minutes.

3. Add the broccoli rabe and water. Cover and cook until the leaves are wilted and the stems are crisp-tender, about 5 minutes.

4. Sprinkle with the orange zest, chile powder, and salt. Toss well. Cover and cook, stirring once or twice, until tender, 3 to 4 minutes.

Per 1-cup serving: 72 calories • 5g protein • 4g fat (0.5g saturated) • 3.5g fiber 159mg calcium • 36mg vitamin C • 6g carbohydrate • 120mg sodium

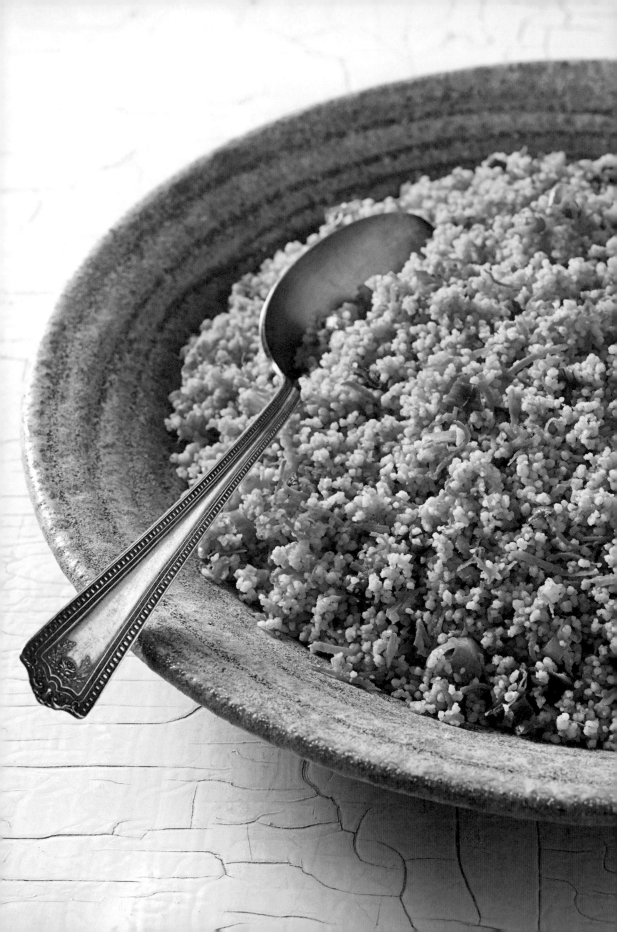

Choose-Your-Own Couscous

Hands-On Time: 5 minutes • **Total Time:** 15 minutes • **Makes:** 4 servings

You can easily make couscous in single-serving amounts. Start with ¼ cup dry couscous, 5 tablespoons water, ¼ teaspoon oil, and a pinch of salt and pepper; scale back the add-ins, too. If you've never had whole-wheat couscous before, you'll be pleasantly surprised for two reasons: It tastes like regular couscous, but it has the bonus of 50 percent more fiber.

Fat Releasers
Olive oil,
black pepper,
couscous

1¼ cups water

1 teaspoon extra-virgin olive oil

¼ teaspoon fine sea salt

Large pinch of black pepper

1 cup whole-wheat couscous

ADD-IN (optional; see below)

1. In a small saucepan, combine the water, oil, salt, and pepper and bring to a boil.

2. Remove from the heat and stir in the couscous and ADD-IN (if using). Cover and let stand for 5 minutes. Fluff with a fork.

▶ ADD-INS

Lemony Spinach: 1 cup coarsely shredded baby spinach, grated zest of ½ lemon, and 2 teaspoons fresh lemon juice.
Fat Releasers: Spinach, lemon

Garlic-Herb: 1 small grated garlic clove (use a citrus zester), ½ cup chopped parsley, and ½ cup chopped fresh basil
Fat Releasers: Garlic, parsley, basil

Green & Orange: 3 chopped scallions, ¾ cup finely grated carrots, 2 teaspoons grated orange zest, and 2 tablespoons fresh orange juice
Fat Releasers: Scallions, orange

Typical ½-cup serving: 180 calories • 7g protein • 1.5g fat (0g saturated) • 6g fiber 20mg calcium • 0mg vitamin C • 37g carbohydrate • 145mg sodium

Toasted Brown Basmati Rice with Scallions

Hands-On Time: 5 minutes • **Total Time:** 55 minutes • **Makes:** 6 servings

Amylopectin is a type of starch that makes certain rices (like Arborio or sushi rice) creamy or sticky. It's the bad-carb part of rice. Luckily, basmati rice is exceptionally low in amylopectin; and when you eat *brown* basmati, you're also getting a helping of fiber. If you have leftovers, freeze them in ½-cup portions and save for making rice salads or throwing into soups.

Fat Releasers
Olive oil, scallions, garlic, brown rice

1 **tablespoon olive oil**
1 **bunch scallions, chopped**
1 **clove garlic, minced**
1 **cup brown basmati rice**
2 **cups water**
¼ **teaspoon fine sea salt**
SEASONING (optional, opposite)

1. In a medium saucepan, heat the oil over medium-high heat. Add the scallions and garlic. Stir until fragrant, about 45 seconds. Stir in the rice to coat. Continue stirring for 2 minutes to lightly toast.

2. Add the water, salt, and SEASONING (if using). Bring to a boil over high heat. Reduce to a low simmer, stir once, tightly cover, and cook for 40 minutes. Remove from the heat and let sit, covered, for 10 minutes. Fluff with a fork.

Per ½-cup serving: 132 calories • 3g protein • 3.5g fat (0.5g saturated) • 2g fiber 18mg calcium • 4mg vitamin C • 25g carbohydrate • 102mg sodium

▶ SEASONINGS

Garlic-Pepper: Add 2 extra garlic cloves when you cook the scallions.
Add ½ teaspoon coarsely ground black pepper when you add the salt.
Fat Releasers: Garlic, black pepper
Per ½-cup serving: 134 calories • 3g protein • 3.5g fat (0.5g saturated) • 2g fiber
21mg calcium • 4mg vitamin C • 25g carbohydrate • 103mg sodium

Orange-Thyme: Add 1 teaspoon dried thyme and the grated zest
of ½ orange when you add the salt.
Fat Releasers: Thyme, orange
Per ½-cup serving: 134 calories • 3g protein • 3.5g fat (0.5g saturated) • 2g fiber
23mg calcium • 6mg vitamin C • 25g carbohydrate • 103mg sodium

Spicy Yellow: Add 1 teaspoon turmeric, ½ teaspoon ground cumin, and
⅛ teaspoon cayenne pepper when you add the salt.
Fat Releaser: Cayenne pepper
Per ½-cup serving: 135 calories • 3g protein • 3.5g fat (0.5g saturated) • 2g fiber
20mg calcium • 4mg vitamin C • 25g carbohydrate • 103mg sodium

Coconut-Basil: Add 2 tablespoons unsweetened shredded coconut to the
pan when you add the rice to toast it. Stir in ¼ cup shredded fresh basil at the end.
Fat Releasers: Coconut, basil
Per ½-cup serving: 144 calories • 3g protein • 4.5g fat (1.5g saturated) • 2g fiber
22mg calcium • 5mg vitamin C • 25g carbohydrate • 103mg sodium

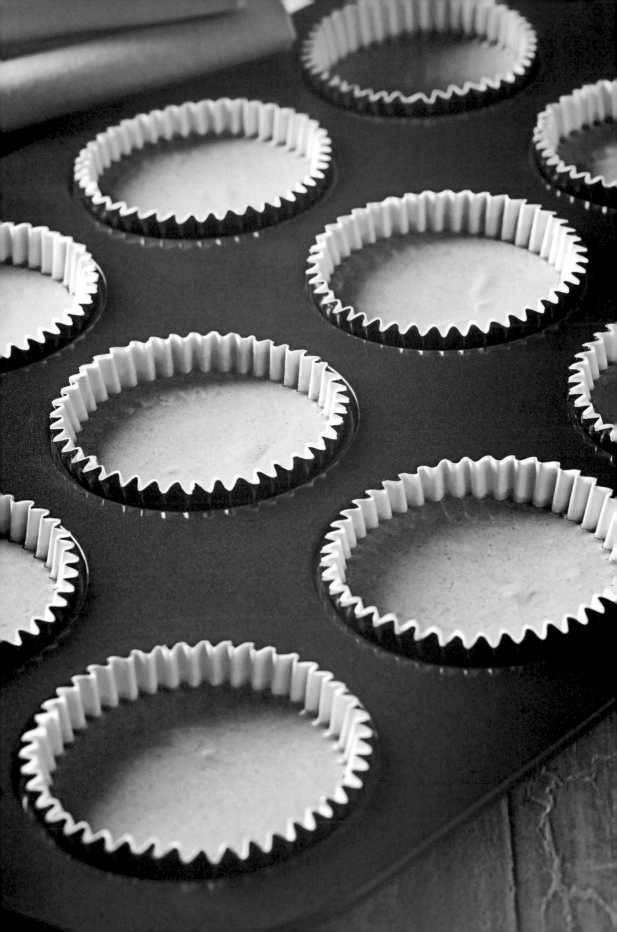

Milk Chocolate Cheesecakelets

Hands-On Time: 15 minutes • **Total Time:** 45 minutes + chilling time
Makes: 10 servings

You can pack these in the freezer for future enjoyment. Let them come back to room temperature and they'll be just as creamy as they were when they came out of the oven.

Fat Releasers
Almonds, cream cheese, yogurt, egg, honey, cocoa

- 1 ounce natural (skin-on) almonds (about 20)
- 8 ounces ⅓-less-fat cream cheese (Neufchâtel)
- 8 ounces 0% Greek yogurt
- 2 egg whites
- ¼ cup + 2 teaspoons honey
- 1 tablespoon unsweetened cocoa powder
- 1 teaspoon vanilla extract

1. Position a rack in the middle of the oven. Preheat the oven to 350°F.

2. Toast the almonds in a shallow pan in the oven or in a dry skillet until crisp and fragrant, 3 to 5 minutes. Finely chop.

3. Fill a rimmed baking sheet with about ¼ inch of water and set a 12-cup muffin tin in the water. Line 10 cups of the tin with foil cupcake cups (with paper liners) and evenly divide the almonds among them (about 1 teaspoon each).

4. In a food processor, combine the cream cheese, yogurt, egg whites, honey, cocoa powder, and vanilla. Blend well and divide the batter among the muffin cups.

5. Bake until set but still a little loose, about 30 minutes. Remove from the oven and let cool in the water bath. Refrigerate until well chilled and set.

Per 1-cakelet serving: 122 calories • 6g protein • 6.5g fat (3g saturated) • 0.5g fiber 50mg calcium • 0mg vitamin C • 11g carbohydrate • 96mg sodium

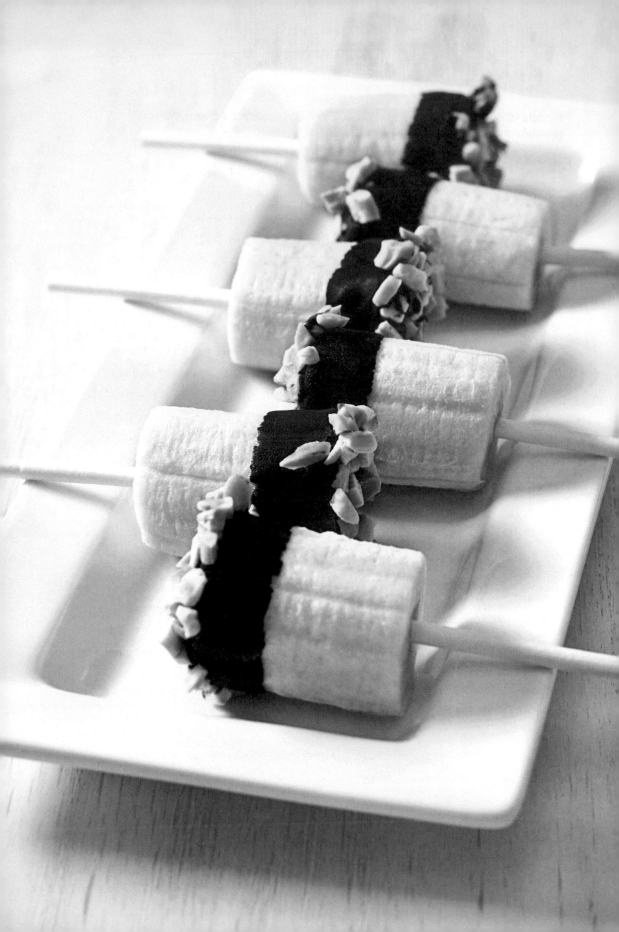

Banana Bonbons

Hands-On Time: 10 minutes • **Total Time:** 10 minutes + freezing time
Makes: 4 servings

Only my family and close friends know this about me (until now, I guess), but I often will eat dessert before the main meal. And these treats are some of my favorites. They are so easy to make, you can double or triple the recipe if you're having company. If you've made them well ahead, let them sit at room temperature for about 30 minutes to soften or they'll be too hard to bite into.

Fat Releasers
Chocolate, nut/olive oil, peanuts

2 bananas

1½ ounces semisweet or bittersweet chocolate

1 teaspoon expeller-pressed nut oil (such as almond) or extra-light olive oil

3 tablespoons finely chopped raw peanuts (¾ ounce)

1. Line a small pan with parchment paper or a nonstick liner. Cut each banana into 6 or 8 equal pieces. Stick a toothpick or lollipop stick into the end of each piece, place in the pan, and put in the freezer to freeze solid.

2. Place the chocolate in a glass 1-cup measure and microwave in 30-second increments, stirring between each, until melted. Add the oil and stir until very smooth.

3. Place the peanuts in a small bowl. Dip the banana pieces halfway into the melted chocolate and shake off the excess. Dip just the end of the banana in the peanuts.

4. Return the bananas to the freezer for 15 minutes to set the chocolate, then store in an airtight container in the freezer. Have 3 large or 4 small bonbons per serving (depending on how you cut the banana).

Per 3- or 4-piece serving: 145 calories • 3g protein • 7.5g fat (3g saturated) 3g fiber • 13mg calcium • 5mg vitamin C • 20g carbohydrate • 2mg sodium

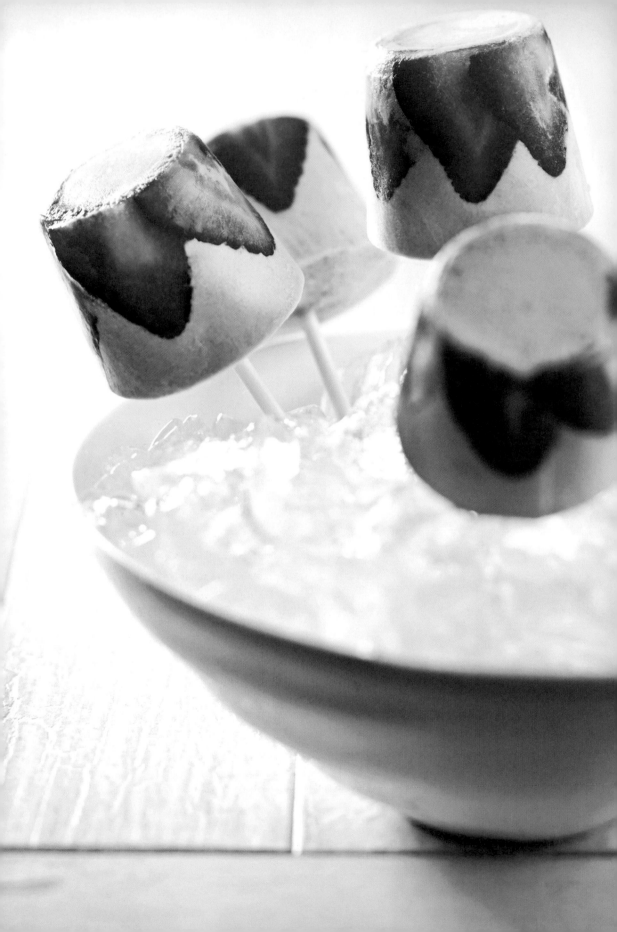

Strawberry Poplets

Hands-On Time: 15 minutes • **Total Time:** 15 minutes + freezing time
Makes: 6 servings

High in vitamin C and calcium, these pops weigh in at less than 100 calories, making them a good choice for a snack. You can easily halve or double the recipe. Store the frozen pops, still in their paper cups, in an airtight container. Or if you're serving these to a group of people, here's a cute presentation: Place half an apple, cut-side down, in a bowl. Push the lollipop sticks into the apple (like a flower arrangement) and cover the apple with ice to hide it and to keep the pops cool.

Fat Releasers
Strawberries, ricotta cheese, honey

1 **quart strawberries**
1 **cup part-skim ricotta cheese**
1 **tablespoon + 1 teaspoon honey**
Pinch of ground allspice

1. Thinly slice enough strawberries lengthwise to get 36 slices for decoration.
2. Halve the remaining strawberries and place them in a food processor. Add the ricotta, honey, and allspice to the processor and puree until smooth.
3. Line the sides of six 3-ounce paper cups with 6 strawberry slices apiece, overlapping slightly. Spoon 2 heaping tablespoons of the strawberry-ricotta mixture into each cup.
4. Place in the freezer until firm enough to insert a lollipop stick into the top, about 2 hours. Freeze until firm, 2 hours longer.
5. With a pair of thin-bladed scissors, make a small cut in the top of each paper cup and carefully peel it away. Serve immediately.

Per 1 pop serving: 94 calories • 5g protein • 3.5g fat (2g saturated) • 1.5g fiber 124mg calcium • 42mg vitamin C • 11g carbohydrate • 53mg sodium

Fudgy Mocha Brownies

Hands-On Time: 10 minutes • **Total Time:** 30 minutes • **Makes:** 16 servings

Even though these brownies have been given a significant health make-over (all good fats, no cholesterol), they're still fudgy and yummy. Luckily, they freeze very well, so you don't have to worry about the batch going stale. You can let the brownies come to room temp if you want, but they're pretty good straight from the freezer.

Fat Releasers
Cocoa, flaxseed, honey, egg, nut/olive oil

- ¾ cup white whole-wheat flour
- ½ cup unsweetened cocoa powder
- ¼ cup flaxseed meal
- 2 tablespoons turbinado sugar
- 1 teaspoon espresso powder
- ¾ teaspoon baking powder
- ¼ teaspoon baking soda
- ¼ teaspoon fine sea salt
- ¾ cup honey
- ½ cup expeller-pressed nut oil (such as almond) or extra-light olive oil
- 1 teaspoon vanilla extract
- 2 egg whites
- 2 tablespoons water
- Fresh raspberries, for garnish (optional)

1. Preheat the oven to 350°F. Lightly oil an 8- or 9-inch-square baking pan.
2. In a large bowl, whisk together the flour, cocoa, flaxseed meal, sugar, espresso powder, baking powder, baking soda, and salt.
3. Add the honey, oil, vanilla, egg whites, and water. Stir until just combined. Do not overmix.
4. Scrape the batter into the prepared pan. Bake until a wooden pick inserted in the center comes out clean, 15 to 18 minutes.
5. Let cool in the pan on a wire rack. Cut into 16 squares. Set aside any you are planning to serve right away. Spread the remainder out on a baking sheet and freeze. When frozen solid, pack into an airtight freezer container.

Per 1-brownie serving: 153 calories • 2g protein • 8g fat (1g saturated) 2g fiber • 18mg calcium • 0mg vitamin C • 21g carbohydrate • 94mg sodium

Chapter

7

"I love to exercise. I just ran a 5K and take Zumba classes regularly. I'd love to try something new."

—DIANE ROHAN,
LOST 11 POUNDS

Fat Release Workout

Did you know a simple 12-minute routine can seriously up your fat burn? Get ready to move!

R

Remember how the wrong kinds of exercise can help you hold on to fat? Well, here you'll learn exactly how to move to release it. The exercises are simple and straightforward and can be done at home. All the basic Fat Release Moves use your body as the weight, so you don't have to invest money in expensive equipment that sits around collecting dust in the corner. And because you are the weight, your "gym" can travel with you anywhere to be used at any time!

I suggest that you do the Fat Release Workout first thing in the morning. Why? Well, besides it being a great way to wake up your body and start your day off burning fat, it's also part of a philosophy about work and life that I try to follow every day: Do the hardest things first. Not that the workout is hard—we've made it doable for all levels of fitness, I promise! But taking the time to properly care for yourself, and finding time to move every day, is hard for many people. Doing the routine first thing in the morning gets it done and off your must-do list. And research has shown that those who exercise at home are more likely to maintain their weight loss—and their routines.

Run through this 12-minute workout and you start the day with a feeling of accomplishment that you can carry throughout the rest of your day. Everything else you need to do just feels easier from then on!

● DO I HAVE TO?

A brief word to the nonexercisers among you, to the people who ask, Can I just eat the food and forgo the fitness? You *can* lose weight just following the diet plan in this book. (In fact, we asked our test team to follow their normal exercise routine—proving that you can indeed see incredible results simply by changing your eating habits.) So if it feels to you like it's just too much to tackle a new diet and a new exercise regimen at the same time, then you can choose to approach the Digest Diet your own way. You can incorporate the workout after or at any stage during the plan that feels most comfortable to you. My preference, of course, is that you follow the plan as outlined for maximum fat release and success.

> Crafting **a lifestyle that you can follow and enjoy** is the key to your individual success.

But my preferences aren't what matters here: Crafting a lifestyle that you can follow and enjoy is the key to your individual success. Only you know what you can do and what is beyond your present reach. However . . . this is *not* a pass on getting moving.

Whether you follow the exercise plan to a T or not, I do ask you to focus on moving more, walking more, and sitting less each day. I want you to stand up for your health rather than sit down and settle for less.

With that in mind, I've created little reminders in the menu plans in Chapter 5 so that in addition to doing the

Fat Release Workout, you'll get several bursts of activity in. Whether that means hitting the ground (or wall) and giving yourself 20 good push-ups or getting up and walking around your office or home, you just have to do it. Remember that old expression "Use it or lose it"? Well, I'm a firm believer that we have to keep moving to signal to our bodies that we are worth keeping around longer. So give yourself that gift, no matter how you decide to "wrap it," and have some fun adding more movement into each day.

● THE BASICS: EXERCISE TO RELEASE FAT

As we mentioned in Chapter 4, high-intensity interval training, or HIIT, is a great way to jump-start fat burning, develop lean muscle, and ward off unwanted pounds. (Conveniently for us, this type of exercise takes far less time than slogging through a marathon cardio session!) That's why it's at the heart of the Fat Release Workout. We've combined strength training, walking, and HIIT into a daily movement plan to take advantage of the findings of the latest research and put you on the road to a stronger, slimmer, healthier body.

Walking: Researchers from Duke University determined that walking 12 miles per week helps to ward off belly fat. You'll see in the Fat Release Workout Calendar (page 245) that for the first four days of the plan, you walk for 45 to 60 minutes. On Day 5, you begin the Fat Release Workout. To fully take the most advantage of the fat-burning zone created by it, you do a 20-minute walk (about one mile) afterward. On days when you don't do the Fat Release Workout, you'll walk for 45 to 60 minutes (for the first two

WHAT IF I'M TOO BIG TO MOVE COMFORTABLY?

A number of you will be at a starting weight that makes doing the workouts, even the walking portion, difficult and even painful. Don't pile blame, guilt, or anything negative on yourself because of this. That's just added emotional weight that you don't deserve or need. We all begin where we are . . . with what we can do. You can and will lose weight if you only eat the foods on the Digest Diet. Do what you can do to simply move a little more each day.

When you've lost enough weight to begin walking for 5 to 10 minutes at a time, do it. Or if you love to dance, just put on some music and bop around your living room. (One of our test team members, Adrienne, began each day with an hour of dancing around her home to her favorite music.)

After that, add in some of the 1-Minute Activity Bursts from pages 256–257. Week to week, add on another 5 to 10 minutes to your walk or other fun activity. When you're ready for more of a challenge, try the Fat Release Workout on page 246, and then add that to your daily movement repertoire. Bit by bit, step by step, it will get easier and you will get stronger, healthier, and fitter.

weeks of the plan) and for 60 minutes during the last week, Finish Strong. Remember, you do not have to do the walking all at once; it's perfectly acceptable to break it up into "bite-size" segments if you need to.

Strength training: On Day 5, you'll start to work in a simple combination of exercises that you likely already know (or won't find hard to learn). These moves hit all of the major muscle groups, including thighs, butt, chest, and abs, and some of those highly visible ones like the arms. The workout will help you become fit and strong and prepare your body from head to toe. Fitness professional Matthew Schwartz has suggested ways to make each move harder if you need a challenge—just be sure you're strong enough to advance so that you don't injure yourself.

High-intensity interval training (HIIT): The strength-training routine—the 12-Minute Fat Release Workout—has been designed to incorporate the fat releasing twist: HIIT. What makes the HIIT portion of the workout so successful? You'll do short bursts of activity, followed by equally short rest periods. This method keeps your muscles guessing and keeps you in fat-burning mode even after you've finished the workout. The Fat Release Workout At-a-Glance chart (page 247) will walk you through each round of exercises, each circuit, and explain how many repetitions to perform as well as when to rest. You'll do the Fat Release Workout three days a week.

To take advantage of the fat-burning power of the HIIT workout, do it first thing in the morning. (If you're not a morning person, don't worry—it's better to do the workout anytime than not at all!)

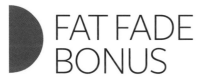

FAT FADE BONUS

Keep those muscles fired up and burning calories by **sprinkling in three to five 1-Minute Activity Bursts throughout the day,** in addition to your normal workout. See pages 256–257 for some great suggestions.

WORKOUT CALENDAR

WEEK #1
DAY 1: Walk 45–60 minutes

DAY 2: Walk 45–60 minutes

DAY 3: Walk 45–60 minutes

DAY 4: Walk 45–60 minutes

DAY 5: Fat Release Workout + 20-minute walk

DAY 6: Walk 45–60 minutes

DAY 7: REST

WEEK #2
DAY 8: Fat Release Workout + 20-minute walk

DAY 9: Walk 45–60 minutes

DAY 10: Fat Release Workout + 20-minute walk

DAY 11: Walk 45–60 minutes

DAY 12: Fat Release Workout + 20-minute walk

DAY 13: Walk 45–60 minutes

DAY 14: REST

WEEK #3
DAY 15: Fat Release Workout (reverse order) + 20-minute walk

DAY 16: Walk 60 minutes

DAY 17: Fat Release Workout (reverse order) + 20-minute walk

DAY 18: Walk 60 minutes

DAY 19: Fat Release Workout (reverse order) + 20-minute walk

DAY 20: Walk 60 minutes

DAY 21: REST

● THE ▼ FAT RELEASE WORKOUT

Remember the 2-for-1 workout we promised in Chapter 4? This is it. You'll ramp up your heart rate and stoke your fat-burning furnaces by performing the exercises quickly with little rest in between. This combination of muscle building and aerobic intervals will fuel your fat release better than either approach on its own.

For each HIIT circuit at right, take about two minutes to do the exercises in the order listed, from top to bottom, then rest for one minute. For example, circuit #1 starts with six to eight chair squats, followed by six to eight push-ups, six to eight more chair squats, six to eight step-ups, and so forth. (See the following pages for photos and detailed descriptions of all exercises.) Repeat the process for circuits #2, #3, and #4, aiming to complete each circuit in two minutes and taking one minute to catch your breath in between. Your heart rate will pick up and your muscles will feel the burn. And in no time flat, you'll be done.

To keep increasing your fat burn, challenge yourself to do more reps in the same amount of time. For example, once eight reps becomes easy, try ten reps of the moves in each two-minute circuit. For an added challenge on Week 3, do the Fat Release Workout in reverse order—start with circuit #4 and work backward to circuit #1. For more ideas on how to progress, see the move descriptions on pages 248–255.

FAT RELEASE WORKOUT AT-A-GLANCE

CIRCUIT #1

1. Squat
2. Push-ups
3. Squats
4. Step-ups
5. Squats
6. Dips
7. Squats

CIRCUIT #2

1. Push-ups
2. Step-ups
3. Push-ups
4. Dips
5. Push-ups
6. Squats
7. Push-ups

CIRCUIT #3

1. Step-ups
2. Dips
3. Step-ups
4. Push-ups
5. Step-ups
6. Squats
7. Step-ups

CIRCUIT #4

1. Dips
2. Squats
3. Dips
4. Push-ups
5. Dips
6. Step-ups
7. Dips

▶ Do 6–8 repetitions of each exercise. For step-ups, do 6–8 reps with each leg.

▶ Complete each circuit in 2 minutes; rest 60 seconds between circuits.

MASTER THE MOVE:
BASIC SQUAT

Muscles Worked:
Butt, thighs, abs

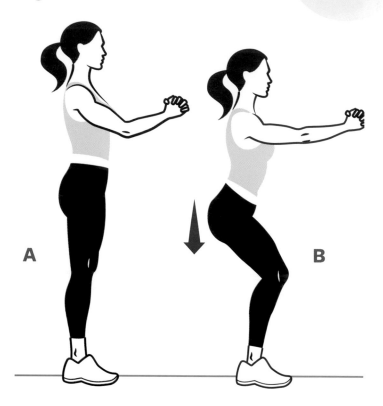

A. Stand with your feet hip-width apart and hands clasped at chest level or on your hips.

B. Bend your legs and squat slightly as if sitting in a chair, keeping your back straight, your knees behind your toes, and your heels flat on the floor. Return to the starting position to complete the move. Perform 6 to 8 reps.

WORK IT HARDER:
ALMOST-SITTING SQUAT

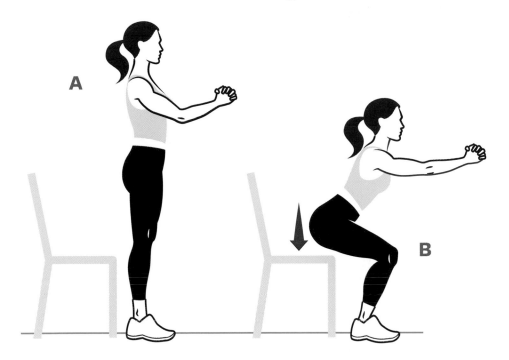

A. Stand in front of a chair with your feet hip-width apart and hands clasped at chest level.

B. With your heels flat on the floor and keeping your back straight, bend your legs and slowly lower your butt until it's nearly touching the chair's seat, but don't sit down. Keep your arms extended in front of you for balance. Return to the starting position to complete the move. Do 10 to 12 reps.

MAX IT OUT:
JUMPING SQUATS

Do the basic squat (opposite), but as you extend your legs to stand, jump straight up, trying to land with a little bend in the knees to cushion your landing before going back into squat position. Do 10 to 12 reps.

Note: If you have knee or back problems, ask your doctor if this exercise is okay for you.

MASTER THE MOVE:
WALL PUSH-UP

Muscles Worked: Abs, back, chest, arms

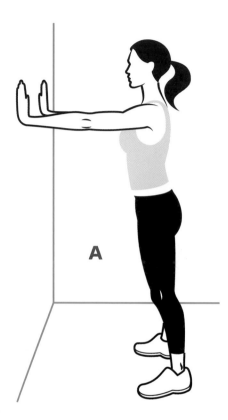

A

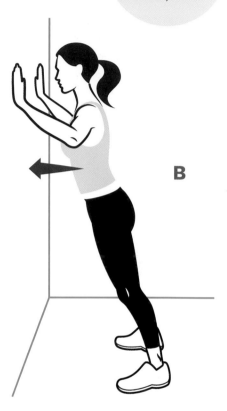

B

A. Stand facing a wall with your feet hip-width apart. Place your palms on the wall at shoulder height and width.

B. Keeping your feet in place, your stomach firm, and your back straight, bend your arms to slowly lower your body toward the wall. If you can, let your chest touch the wall. Extend and straighten your arms to complete the move. Do 6 to 8 reps.

WORK IT HARDER:
CHAIR PUSH-UP

A. Using a sturdy chair, get into a push-up position, extending your arms with your palms on the seat and your legs extended behind you. Your body should form a straight line from your head to your heels.

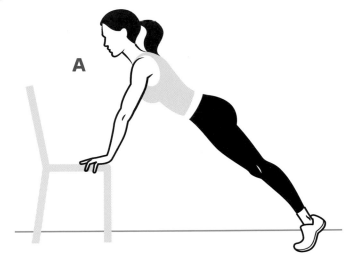

B. Keeping your stomach firm, your back straight, and your elbows tucked near your sides, bend your arms until your chest nearly touches the seat. Extend and straighten your arms to complete the move. Do 10 to 12 reps.

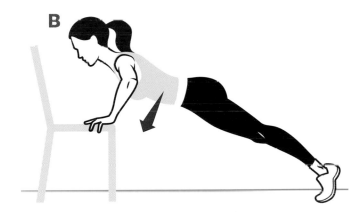

MAX IT OUT:
CLASSIC PUSH-UP

Get into a push-up position with your arms extended, palms on the floor, and legs long and straight behind you. Keeping your stomach firm, your back straight, and your elbows tucked near your sides, bend your arms until your chest nearly touches the floor. Extend your arms to complete the move. If you want an even tougher challenge, try lifting your right leg off the ground for half of the reps, then your left leg off of the ground for the remainder of the reps. Do 10 to 12 reps.

MASTER THE MOVE:
BASIC STEP-UP

Muscles Worked: Thighs, butt, calves

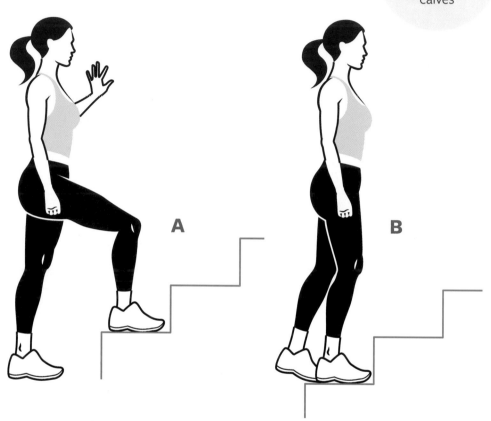

A

B

A. Stand in front of a low step or at the base of a staircase, using a handrail or wall for balance, if necessary. Place your right foot on the first stair.

B. Step up and tap your left foot lightly on the stair. Keeping your right foot on the stair, step down with your left leg to complete the move. Do 6 to 8 reps with each leg.

WORK IT HARDER:
2-STEP STEP-UP

A

B

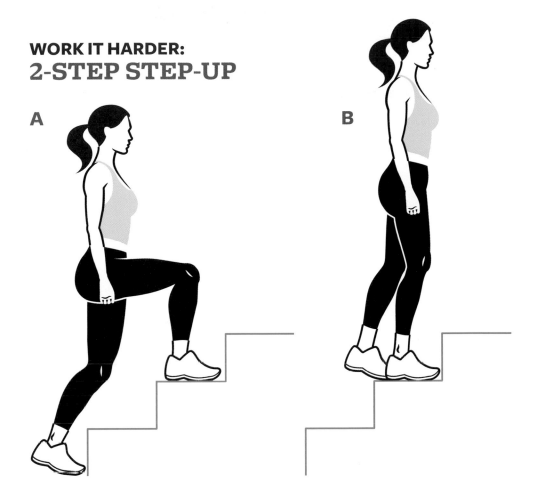

A. Stand in front of a low step or at the base of a staircase. Place your right foot on the second stair.

B. Step up and tap your left foot lightly on the second stair. Keeping your right foot on the stair, step down with your left leg to complete the move. Do 10 to 12 reps with each leg.

MAX IT OUT:
WEIGHT-FOR-IT STEP-UP

Stand in front of a low step or at the base of a staircase holding a full water bottle in each hand (or hold 5- to 10-pound hand weights, if you have them). Place your right foot on the second stair. Step up and tap your left foot lightly on the second stair. Keeping your right foot on the stair, step down with your left leg to complete the move. Do 10 to 12 reps with each leg.

**Muscles
Worked:**
Abs, shoulders,
back, chest,
arms

MASTER THE MOVE:
CLASSIC DIP

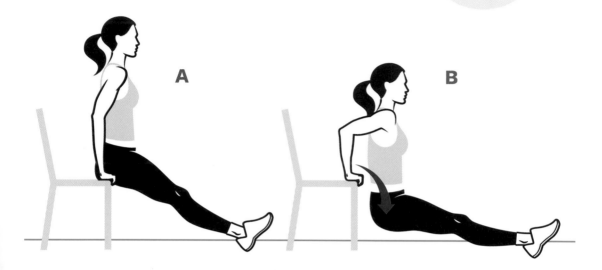

A. Sit in a sturdy, armless chair with your feet flat on the floor. Place your palms on the edge of the seat beside your hips and extend your legs so that only your heels are on the floor.

B. Walk your heels forward until your butt is just in front of the chair and you're supporting your body weight with your arms. Keeping your elbows pointed behind you, bend your arms to lower your body about 6 inches. Extend and straighten your arms to complete the move. Do 6 to 8 reps.

WORK IT HARDER:
LEG-RAISED DIP

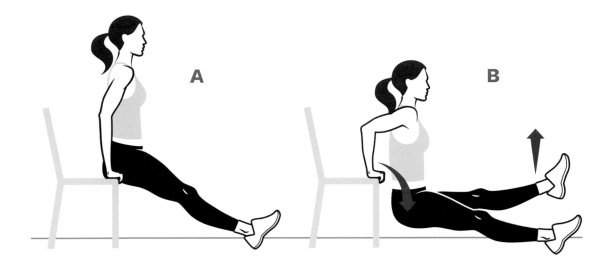

A. Sit in a sturdy, armless chair with your feet flat on the floor. Place your palms on the edge of the seat beside your hips and extend your legs so that only your heels are on the floor.

B. Walk your heels forward until your butt is just in front of the chair and you're supporting your body weight with your arms. Raise your left leg about 12 inches off the floor. Keeping your elbows pointed behind you, bend your arms to lower your body about 6 inches. Extend and straighten your arms to complete the move. Do 5 dips with your left leg raised and 5 dips with your right leg raised.

MAX IT OUT:
DOUBLE-CHAIR DIP

Sit in a sturdy, armless chair facing another chair. Place your palms on the edge of the seat beside your hips and extend your legs so that your heels are on the seat of the second chair. Slowly move forward until your butt is just in front of the chair and you're supporting your body weight with your arms. Keeping your elbows pointed behind you, bend your arms to lower your body about 6 inches. Extend and straighten your arms to complete the move. Do 10 to 12 reps.

● 1-MINUTE ACTIVITY BURSTS!

I've discussed the importance of getting more spontaneous physical activity into your day. And it may seem ironic to "plan" for that activity, but that's what you'll do here, just to get started. I want you to move more and enjoy doing so. All of the ideas below are simple ways to get you started living this way and creating a new mind-set toward staying active. Do these activities for one minute. Strive to do three throughout the day in the first two stages of the diet and five throughout the day from then on. Hey, the more bursts of activity you can add to the day, the healthier you'll be and the more fat you'll release!

Push-ups: Hit the ground and give yourself 20 (or do push-ups against a wall).

Stair climb: Stride upstairs two at a time.

Jumping jacks: Pretend you're a kid again!

Dance: Do it around your living room—just turn on some music and go.

Mountain climbers: Get into a push-up position. Bring one knee in toward the chest with your foot on the floor; extend the other leg straight behind you. Keeping your hands on the floor, your butt low, and your back straight, "jump" up and switch feet in the air so that your opposite leg is now bent. Continue to jump and alternate legs, almost like sprinting in place.

Burpees: Stand with your feet hip-width apart. Bend your knees and lower your body, placing your hands palms down on the floor on the outside of either foot. Jump your legs back so that they're extended and you're in a classic push-up position. Then jump your legs back into the squat position, and as you return to standing, jump straight into the air and land with slightly bent knees in the starting position.

Walking lunge: Need to pick up something from across the room? Lunge over to get it. Step forward with your right foot, then bend both legs so that the right knee is at a 90-degree angle and the left knee nearly touches the floor. Straighten, keeping abs tight, and step forward with the left foot to bring your legs together. Repeat with the opposite leg, then continue alternating legs as you step forward. Walking this way won't win you any races, but you'll be working nearly every lower body muscle as you go.

Bicycle: A recent study found that this gym-class favorite is one of the most effective abs exercises out there. It gets your heart pumping, too. Lie on your back with your feet flat on the floor, gently supporting your head with your hands. Raise both legs until your shins are parallel with the floor. With your abs tight, straighten your left leg and draw your left elbow across your body toward your right knee. Then do the opposite—straighten your right leg and draw your right elbow toward your left knee. Alternate back and forth as if you're pedaling a bike.

Chapter

8

"If you get off track, this
plan helps you get back to a
healthy way of eating.
For that I am grateful!"

—ANNETTE PROCIDA,
LOST 11 POUNDS

Losing More and Keeping It Off

Here's how to use the Digest Diet to reach your goal weight and maintain it. You'll cultivate the top habits that keep you slim for life.

First, before you do anything else, you should reach around and pat yourself on the back for completing the past three weeks of the Digest Diet. Anyone who has ever battled with being overweight knows that it can be a difficult ride that requires focus, dedication, and commitment to see it through to the end.

Though I've tried to create a weight-loss experience that brings a full measure of enjoyment, laughter, and fun to each day, I know that it's your hard work that ultimately translates into success. Congratulate yourself now, whether you've achieved your goal weight or not, as you're making several life-affirming, health-promoting changes that give you a solid foundation for the future.

So what happens now? If you still have more weight to lose, don't worry. Remember, being overweight is not a failing, it's just excess fat. And you now have great tools at your disposal for releasing any extra stores you might still have. Your success can and will continue. Now you just have to adjust your thinking a bit: to slow and steady wins the race.

Compare your journey to a running course. If you have 5 to 10 pounds to lose, that's like a 50-yard dash. You can sprint through it, lose the weight in a short time, and then you're at the finish line. Twenty-five to 50 pounds? Well, that's more like a half-marathon: You need to train consistently and plan ahead, and you'll be in fighting shape over the course of weeks or months, depending on your individual body. For those who have 50 or even more than 100 pounds to lose: Yes, it's a marathon, but you have all the strength it takes to hit that last mile marker.

If you followed this plan, you started strong and made good headway in the first 21 days, while establishing a foundation of healthy eating and fat releasing habits, like moving more and laughing every day. Now you have to pace yourself, surround yourself with support, and pride yourself in taking every step, whether it's a large leap or a small stride. Expecting too much too soon is actually demotivating and detrimental to what you want to accomplish long-term. Follow the precepts of the Digest Diet, together with the advice in this chapter on maintenance, and you can smile your way to the finish line! Here's how.

● IF YOU WANT TO LOSE
10 TO 20 POUNDS

Follow this strategy:

Step 1: Repeat the Fade Away portion of the menu plan for 10 days (pages 126–135).

Step 2: Follow that with one week in Finish Strong (pages 136–142).

Step 3: If you haven't reached your goal weight by then, repeat another week of Finish Strong.

Step 4: Throughout, make sure to keep up your activity. Do the daily Fat Release Workouts in the mornings and add 5 to 10 minutes to your daily walking each week. Top out at 90 minutes—more than that isn't realistic for most of us. And remember, these can be broken up into 5-, 10-, or 20-minute sessions throughout the day; you don't have to walk it all at once.

● IF YOU WANT TO LOSE
20 TO 50 POUNDS

By now, you've learned that losing weight is not an uphill battle—it's more like a long, steady trek. If you aim to shed this range of pounds, the journey could take weeks or months, depending on factors like your individual metabolism and how much movement you build into your days. The key is to strive for that middle place, where you move in the right direction more often than not. The more time you spend eating and living in a health-promoting, joy-fulfilling way, the more likely you will stay at your goal weight permanently.[1] (For more information, see "Keeping It Off" later in this chapter.)

Option 1: Do over. If you're comfortable doing so, you can repeat Fade Away and Finish Strong until you reach your goal weight. At this stage in the process, you can expect to lose around one to three pounds a week.

Option 2: Branch out. If you want to branch out on your own for even more variety, reread the chapters on fat increasers and fat releasers. Then create your own menu plans. You know which foods to eat and why. Use the Fade Away and Finish Strong phases as models, and plan your portions and menus. Use the Fat Releaser Food Lists (pages 96–111) and the Fat Release Recipes (Chapter 6) to

WHY YOU SHOULDN'T REPEAT THE FAST RELEASE PHASE

A number of our test panelists wondered if they could just cycle through the three-week plan repeatedly until reaching their goal weight. Here are my thoughts on why you should wait to repeat Fast Release for at least a month, if not two months.

The calorie levels (1,200) for this first stage of the Digest Diet were designed for very fast weight loss. Research supported the notion of jump-starting your efforts, but its low calorie count encouraged me to limit it to four days. I do not believe in long-term deprivation; that's a mind-set that will push you toward not achieving what you want. Plus, it's not sustainable to eat this way for the long term. Doing this type of jump start for too long might actually boomerang on you: Your body might perceive that it's under threat of deprivation and decide to hold tighter to its fat stores.

If you have more weight to lose, repeat cycling through Fade Away and Finish Strong. Wait at least a month to throw in a Fast Release. And don't do it more frequently than four times a year if this is a longer journey for you.

get you started. You'll also find guidelines for how to mix and match recipes in Chapter 6 (see pages 148–151).

All of the recipes in this book come with calorie counts and nutrition information. Feel free to mix and match them to your tastes and preferences, while keeping within a reasonable calorie limit (see "Keep Watch on Your Calorie Intake," page 264).

Choose lean and green first. Fill up on nutritious soups and fiber-rich vegetables and grains. Eat three servings of fat-free dairy each day. For your fats, choose MUFAs and omega-3 PUFAs (see page 102). Be sure to include three meals and two snacks in each day (if you are using the Finish Strong phase as your guide, have one dessert a week). Write down your picks and your favorites, and plan out your meals, one week at a time, shopping accordingly.

Keep watch on your calorie intake. Women should aim to eat between 1,400 and 1,600 calories a day; men, 1,600 to 1,800 calories. Don't let more than three hours pass between meals and snacks; this is still a relatively low calorie intake, so you don't want to spike your hunger by going too long between meals.

Fill up on greens. There may be days where you feel hungry eating this level of calories. Perhaps you did an extra-long workout. Maybe you have hormone-induced cravings. Possibly, you're just having a stressful day! During times like these, experiment by upping your intake by another 100 calories. This should not stop you from continuing to lose. Add a large vegetable serving, a hefty salad (no extras here, just stick to veggies and a teaspoon of Digest Diet Vinaigrette), another snack, or a one-cup serving of any of the soups from Chapter 6 to that day's menu.

DIGEST THIS...

A **diet rich in high-fiber foods** now appears to be even better for you: It seems to **protect against not just heart disease but also infectious and respiratory diseases.** In a study of almost 400,000 people, those who ate the most fiber were 22 percent less likely to die during a nine-year period than fiber avoiders. Plus, people who ate more soluble fiber (the type found in fruit, beans, and oats, among other foods) over a five-year period **gained less belly fat**—which, as we know, is the most dangerous fat for health.

Step it up! Step up your exercise routine, and when you perform the 12-Minute Fat Release Workout in Chapter 7, power it up and advance to the next most difficult variation provided. Don't forget to breathe deeply and stay hydrated. Perform the full routine every other day or try SIT instead (see below).

SIT. This acronym does not mean what you think it means. On one of your days off from the Fat Release Workout, challenge yourself to 12 minutes of SIT: sprint interval training. This is another form of high-intensity interval training, and it follows the same basic steps as HIIT but with sprinting/ jogging intervals as your hard/easy periods of cardio. Here's how it works:

First, warm up for about 4 minutes so your muscles are ready for the demands about to be placed on them. Then sprint at your fastest pace for 30 seconds. Actively rest for 30 seconds; slow down to a very slow walk so you can catch your breath. Repeat this sequence six times. You can do it on a treadmill or have fun hitting the corners going around the block: Sprint on one stretch, round the corner, and do the straightaway at a jog, then sprint/jog until you are done. If you don't live on a block, you can alternate it on any stretch of road.

Take another 2 minutes to gradually power down, with shorter bursts (15 seconds) and longer recovery times (45 seconds), and you're done. You have another effective 12-minute workout—and you can extend it if you like, but it's best to keep it to no longer than 16 minutes so you don't overdo it.

Don't forget to stretch after—and don't neglect your warm-up, as you can injure yourself if your body isn't ready for intense work like this.

IF YOU WANT TO LOSE
50 TO 100 POUNDS OR MORE

All of the advice above for those wanting to lose 25-plus pounds applies here, so incorporate it all as you move forward. No matter how long it takes to get there, you can and will get there. Want proof? Simple. You've lost weight when you've focused on doing so, right? Then you can do this now. Along the way, remember these tools:

Read up. Read or reread "If You Want to Lose 20 to 50 Pounds," and follow the eating and exercise advice.

> Take it **one meal, one day, one pound** at a time.

Log it. Keep a notebook—or your mobile phone or laptop, if that's what you prefer— at hand to help you along your way. This is crucial. Use it not only to set your weekly, monthly, and yearly goals but also as a place to keep track of your successes and challenges. Write everything down.

It might also help to keep a visual diary of what you've accomplished—whether it's weekly photos you take of yourself and place in a beautiful album or a video log recording your week's successes and weight lost. When you feel you've hit a plateau or your energy is flagging, you'll have a record on hand to review all that you've accomplished. There's nothing more inspiring than seeing your success!

Take it one pound at a time. If you focus on thinking, "I have 50, or 100, or more pounds to lose," it can be overwhelming. Take it one meal, one day, one pound at a time. Write down what you'd like to specifically accomplish each week, as well as a goal for each month. Don't think reality TV pounds here, either. Keep it simple: one pound this week; five pounds this month. Something that's doable, achievable, and won't stress you out thinking about accomplishing it!

Fill up on life. Often, we "starve" ourselves of fun in our lives but eat until we feel stuffed. What we should be doing instead is to stop at feeling satisfied. This takes time and practice to learn. When it comes to your life, fill it to the brim! If you focus on family, friends, love, and enjoyable activities, food becomes relegated to a much smaller role, and life becomes richer, deeper, and absolutely fuller.

Don't expect too much too soon. Setting too-high expectations for your weekly or monthly weight loss is perhaps as damaging as setting them too low. In either event, you are destined to fail. If the bar is too low ("I will lose one pound each month"), you have little success to motivate you. Set the bar too high ("I want to drop two pounds a day, every day!"), and you likely will end up beating up on yourself for falling short. Instead of moving forward, you'll be stuck close to the start.

This links back to a theme I've tried to weave throughout: finding that middle place. The reality is that you probably will not meet your goals every week. When that happens, move on from it. Start the next meal or the next day by

 LAUGH IT OFF

My sister decided to go on a diet, and that first evening, she phoned me. I could tell her mouth was full, so I asked her what she was eating.

"A cupcake," she mumbled. "I just got on the scale, and it read 149½. I decided that that was no place to start a diet, so I'm rounding it up to 150."

—SHARON E. ASKEGREEN

remembering to take it a pound at a time. You'll get where you need to go.

Reward yourself along the way. Have you wanted to do something special for yourself? Maybe it's spending a whole day unplugged, or maybe it's the dance or music lessons you've always wanted to take.

Well, for every pound lost, put a dollar toward your dream. If you can afford more than that, then give yourself a raise. If it's not money but time that you need, set a half hour aside for each pound lost.

Buddy up. Our test panel noted (and research supports) that doing the diet with a friend, a spouse, or coworkers helped them to stick with the plan and succeed.

It's easier to keep on this journey if you don't walk it alone. Buddy up with a friend, spouse, sister, brother, mother, or cousin and help each other go the distance. You don't have to be in the same city or even the same state to do this, either. Create a by-invitation-only Facebook page with a group of your friends, relatives, or colleagues who also want to lose weight. Or go to readersdigest.com/digestdiet or facebook.com/digestdiet to find ways that *Reader's Digest* can connect you to other Digest Dieters.

● KEEPING IT OFF

It's a depressing statistic: Most people who lose weight don't keep it off long-term. And maybe you're worried about that. But rather than getting discouraged and giving up, I'd like you to shift your perspective a bit.

I prefer to focus on the people who *do* succeed at maintaining their weight loss over the long haul. I looked at what recent research on successful maintainers has revealed. I found it both surprising and reassuring that many of the successful maintainers "were currently older and had been dieting longer" when they found their "stride." A study done at Kings College in London compared the differences between groups of women who were long-term maintainers and those who either stayed obese or regained weight. The maintainers tended to be older women.[2] This is but one factor and one study, but age might be on your side here—as is the hard work from past attempts!

I was surprised by how many studies (including one that reviewed more than 65 years of research) pointed to similar helpful tools over and over again. Put them to work for you!

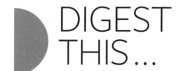

DIGEST THIS...

Yet another reason to play more: It can keep you from working too hard. **Keeping long hours at work may raise your risk of heart disease.** People who regularly worked 11-hour days were almost 70 percent more likely to develop heart disease than those who put in 8-hour days.

THE 8 HABITS OF SUCCESSFUL MAINTAINERS

1. They are physically active each day.

One of the biggest predictors of long-term weight-loss success is physical activity.[3] Remember reading earlier that exercise *alone* isn't a great weight-loss tool? Well, it is a great way to prevent weight gain and preserve lean body mass. The more you move each day and the more fit you become, the better your success will be in keeping the pounds and fat off. But as with everything in the journey, be realistic. Add in activity and exercise gradually, and mix it up.

Aim to progressively increase exercise to five hours per week, as it has been shown to make lifetime maintenance easier.[4] Remember, this can be broken up into different intervals and different types of activity. Those short bouts might just be more effective than big chunks of activity, anyway! Plus, they are easier to commit to.[5]

2. They eat breakfast.

Who'd have thought that something so simple could be so powerful? You know from Chapter 2 that skipping breakfast can derail your weight-loss efforts. Well, the same is true for keeping weight off. Even if all you have time for is a handful of nuts and a piece of fruit, even if you're not particularly hungry in the morning, eat something. Start each day by doing this elemental and simple good thing for yourself (hopefully paired with a 12-minute home workout). It can cause a positive ripple effect throughout the day.

 LAUGH IT OFF

My daughter couldn't muster the willpower to lose unwanted pounds. One day, watching a svelte friend walking up our driveway, she lamented, "Linda's so skinny it makes me sick."

"If it bothers you," I suggested gently, "why don't you do something about it?"

"Good idea, Mom," she replied. Turning to her friend, she called out, "Hey, Linda, have a piece of chocolate cake." —DORIS E. FLETCHER

3. They control their portions.

As I finish writing this book, Thanksgiving has passed and we're running smack into the end-of-year celebrations that come with the holiday season. That means facing a lot of tempting food. Does this mean I decline all treats and desserts? Absolutely not! But it does mean that I control how much I put on my plate. And that's true no matter what the season. Keep it up and you'll keep it off.[6]

> Who'd have thought that something so simple could be so powerful?

4. They make healthy food choices.

You know how to make good food choices: by eating the fresh, whole foods that you've been eating on the Digest Diet. Enjoy any recipes you never got a chance to try in Chapter 6. Continue to balance your plate with your favorite fat releasers. Keep to the "thrive with five" tip (page 83).Those who maintain lost weight generally stick to a diet low in unhealthy fats while high in fiber from fruits, vegetables, and whole grains.

5. They keep track.

Those who succeed self-monitor their food intake and keep track of their weight. They pay attention to their daily behaviors and activities and steer themselves toward healthy ones. Some get on the scale each week. Some track inches lost. Some track steps taken, literally, by wearing a pedometer and writing down how many steps they take each day.

How you decide to keep track is entirely up to you, but write it down. If your device of choice is a pen, a laptop, or a mobile phone, take advantage of the wealth of tools available.

Consider focusing on an issue or area that you feel hasn't been in your control before: whether that's what you're eating or what you're feeling. You can journal about your hopes and dreams. You can jot down all the things you've done that make you laugh, give you joy, or make you happy. Keep a calendar of how long you've succeeded and applaud every day that's passed where you've taken any small measure to take good care of yourself.

> Maintenance **may get easier** over time.

6. They find food-free ways to deal with stress.

I hope that our journey together has showed you the importance of both a positive attitude and in wringing the joy out of each day. We can all afford to take more time away from being a "grown-up" and seek out things that delight us, ignite us, and make us sparkle inside. Give yourself the permission to make doing these things a priority.

If you've been a stress eater in the past, now is the time to explore your personal triggers and defuse them, replacing them with more proactive and caring behaviors. When you're stressed, redouble your commitment to getting seven to eight hours of sleep. Being sleep deprived makes you more sensitive to stress and increases hunger.

When you feel the urge to do something unhealthy, remember to pause to examine the cause. Instead of reaching for a cookie, reach for a friend. If you're angry, walk it off. This simple switching of behaviors can teach you marvelous new ways to cope.

If you are still struggling with any issues that may be

weighing you down emotionally, there's no shame in seeking professional help from a doctor or therapist.

7. They surround themselves with support.

I can't stress this enough: Don't go it alone. And support can't just come from others: You need to set up your household, your day, and your work environment to support you, too. (If you need to, reread the section on Environment on pages 68–74 as a refresher.) That means not bringing junk food into the house if that's a trigger for you. It means planning ahead when it comes to snacking and traveling. It means not letting yourself go so long between meals that you find yourself famished.

Seek out things that **delight you and make you sparkle** inside.

It means deciding each day to take care of you.

8. They believe they can do it.

We have faith in so many things, so why is it that we neglect to believe in the best of ourselves? We see our failings, not our victories. We note what we can't do, not what we have accomplished. We seek out flaws, not our strengths.

I hope that reading this book and continuing to track your progress has helped shift this type of thinking for you. My wish is that you clearly see the amazing miracle that is your body and your life, and that you fully embrace the gift we are all given by simply being here.

Notes

Chapter 1

1. Ryan, R. M., Frederick, C. "On energy, personality, and health: subjective vitality as a dynamic reflection of well-being." *Journal of Personality* 65, no. 3 (1997): 529–65.
2. Sublette, M. E., Ellis, S. P., Geant, A. L., Mann, J. J. "Meta-analysis of the effects of eicosapentaenoic acid (EPA) in clinical trials in depression." *Journal of Clinical Psychiatry,* September 6, 2011.
3. Lee, J. H., O'Keefe, J. H., Lavie, C. J., Marchioli, R., Harris, W. S. "Omega-3 fatty acids for cardioprotection." *Mayo Clinic Proceedings* 83, no. 3 (2011): 324–32.
4. Gleissman, H., Johnsen, J. I., Kogner, P. "Omega-3 fatty acids in cancer, the protectors of good and the killers of evil?" *Experimental Cell Research* 316, no. 8 (May 1, 2010): 1365–73. Epub 2010 Mar 6.

Chapter 2

1. Swinburn, B., Sacks, G., Ravussin, E. "Increased food energy supply is more than sufficient to explain the US epidemic of obesity." *American Journal of Clinical Nutrition* 90, no. 6 (December 2009): 1453–6. Epub 2009 Oct 14.
2. Swithers, S. E., Ogden, S. B., Davidson, T. L. "Fat substitutes promote weight gain in rats consuming high-fat diets." *Behavioral Neuroscience* 125, no. 4 (August 2011): 512–8.
3. Giovannini, M., Agostoni, C., Shamir, R. "Symposium overview: Do we all eat breakfast and is it important?" *Critical Reviews in Food Science and Nutrition* 50, no. 2 (February 2010): 97–99.
4. Tremblay, A., Chaput, J. P. "About unsuspected potential determinants of obesity." *Applied Physiology, Nutrition and Metabolism* 33, no. 4 (August 2008): 791–6.
5. Johnston, C. S. "Strategies for healthy weight loss: from vitamin C to the glycemic response." *Journal of the American College of Nutrition* 24, no. 3 (June 2005): 158–65.
6. Major, G. C., et al. "Multivitamin and dietary supplements, body weight and appetite: results from a cross-sectional and a randomised, double-blind placebo-controlled study." *British Journal of Nutrition* 99, no. 5 (May 2008): 1157–167.
7. Teske, J. A., Billington, C. J., Kuskowski, M. A., and Kotz, C. M. "Spontaneous physical activity protects against fat mass gain." *International Journal of Obesity* (May 24, 2011).

8. Tremblay, A., Therrien, F. "Physical activity and body functionality: Implications for obesity prevention and treatment." *Canadian Journal of Physiology and Pharmacology* 84, no. 2 (February 2006): 149–56.

9. Chaput J. P., Tremblay A. "Does short sleep duration favor abdominal adiposity in children?" *International Journal of Pediatric Obesity* 2, no. 3 (2007): 188–91.

10. Xu, X., Liu, C., Xu, Z., Tzan, K., Zhong, M., Wang, A., Lippmann, M., Chen, L. C., Rajagopalan, S., Sun, Q. "Long-term exposure to ambient fine particulate pollution induces insulin resistance and mitochondrial alteration in adipose tissue." *Toxicological Sciences* 124, no. 1 (November 2011): 88–98. Epub 2011 Aug 27.

11. Kramer, Holly, Cao, G., Dugas, L., Luke, A., Cooper, R., Durazo-Arvizu, R. "Increasing BMI and waist circumference and prevalence of obesity among adults with Type 2 diabetes: the National Health and Nutrition Examination Surveys." *Journal of Diabetes and Its Complications* 24, no. 6 (November–December 2010): 368–74. Epub 2009 Nov 14.

12. Jakicic, J. M. "The effect of physical activity on body weight." *Obesity* 17, supplement no. 3 (December 2009): S34–8.

13. Hopkins, M., Jeukendrup, A., King, N. A., Blundell, J. E. "The relationship between substrate metabolism, exercise and appetite control: does glycogen availability influence the motivation to eat, energy intake or food choice?" *Sports Medicine* 41, no. 6 (June 1, 2011): 507–21.

14. Brock, David W., Chandler-Laney, Paula C., Alvarez, Jessica A., Gower, Barbara. A., Gaesser, Glenn A., and Hunter, Gary R. "Perception of exercise difficulty predicts weight regain in formerly overweight women." *Journal of Obesity* 18, no. 5 (2010): 982–86.

15. Chandler-Laney, P. C., Brock, D. W., Gower, B. A., Alvarez, J. A., Bush, N. C., Hunter, G. R. "Self-reported low vitality, poor mental health, and low dietary restraint are associated with overperception of physical exertion." *Journal of Obesity* 2010; 2010: Epub 2010 207451. Sep 26.

16. See note 12 above.

17. Lindvall, K., Larsson, C., Weinehall, L., Emmelin, M. "Weight maintenance as a tightrope walk—a Grounded Theory study." *BMC Public Health* 10 (2010): 51.

Chapter 3

1. Canoy, D., Wareham, N., Welch, A., Bingham, S., Luben, R., Day, N., Khaw, K. T. "Plasma ascorbic acid concentrations and fat distribution in 19,068 British men and women in the European Prospective Investigation into Cancer and Nutrition Norfolk cohort study." *American Journal of Clinical Nutrition* 82, no. 6 (December 2005): 1203–9.

2. Zemel, M. B., Miller, S. L. "Dietary calcium and dairy modulation of adiposity and obesity risk." *Nutrition Review* 62, no. 4 (April 2004): 125–31.

3. Zemel, M. B. "The role of dairy foods in weight management." *Journal of the American College of Nutrition* 24, supplement no. 6 (December 2005): 537S–46S.

4. Josse, A. R., Tang, J. E., Tarnopolsky, M. A., Phillips, S. M. "Body composition and strength changes in women with milk and resistance exercise." *Medicine and Science in Sports and Exercise* 42, no. 6 (June 2010): 1122–30.

5. Johnston, C. S. "Strategies for healthy weight loss: from vitamin C to the glycemic response." *Journal of the American College of Nutrition* 24, no. 3 (June 2005): 158–65.

6. Van Marken Lichtenbelt, W. D., Mensink, R. P., Westerterp, K. R. "The effect of fat composition of the diet on energy metabolism." *Z Ernahrungswiss* 36, no. 4 (December 1997): 303–5.

7. Mercer, S. W., Trayhurn, P. "Effect of high-fat diets on energy balance and thermogenesis in brown adipose tissue of lean and genetically obese ob/ob mice." *Journal of Nutrition* 117, no. 12 (December 1987): 2147–53.

8. Calder, P. C. "Polyunsaturated fatty acids and inflammation." *Prostaglandins, Leukotrienes, and Essential Fatty Acids* 75, no. 3 (September 2006): 197–202.

9. Assunção, M. L,. Ferreira, H.S., dos Santos, A. F., Cabral, C. R., Jr., Florêncio, T. M. "Effects of dietary coconut oil on the biochemical and anthropometric profiles of women presenting abdominal obesity." *Lipids* 44, no. 7 (July 2009): 593–601. Epub 2009 May 13.

10. Lipoeto, N. I., Agus, Z., Oenzil, F., Wahlqvist, M., Wattanapenpaiboon, N. "Dietary intake and the risk of coronary heart disease among the coconut-consuming Minangkabau in West Sumatra, Indonesia." *Asia Pacific Journal of Clinical Nutrition* 13, no. 4 (2004): 377–84.

11. Wang, L., Lee, I. M., Manson, J. E., Buring, J. E., Sesso, H. D. "Alcohol consumption, weight gain, and risk of becoming overweight in middle-aged and older women." *Archives of Internal Medicine* 170, no. 5 (March 8, 2010): 453–61.

12. Smith, R. R., Hong, J., Harvey, A. E., Lewis, T., Diaz, D., Núñez, N. P. "Ethanol consumption does not promote weight gain in female mice." *Annals of Nutrition and Metabolism* 53, no. 3–4 (2008): 252–9. Epub 2009 Jan 9.

13. Lagouge, M., et al. "Resveratrol improves mitochondrial function and protects against metabolic disease by activating SIRT1 and PGC-1alpha." *Cell* 127, no. 6 (December 15, 2006): 1109–22. Epub 2006 Nov 16.

14. Kondo, T., Kishi, M., Fushimi, T., Kaga, T. "Acetic acid upregulates the expression of genes for fatty-acid oxidation enzymes in liver to suppress body-fat accumulation." *Journal of Agricultural and Food Chemistry* 57, no. 13 (July 8, 2009): 5982–6.

15. Meneguetti, Q.A., Brenzan, M. A., Batista, M. R., Bazotte, R. B., Silva, D. R., Garcia Cortez, D. A. "Biological effects of hydrolyzed quinoa extract from seeds of Chenopodium quinoa Willd." *Journal of Medicinal Food* 14, no. 6 (June 2011): 653–7. Epub 2011 Apr 11.

16. Nemoseck, T. M., Carmody, E. G., Furchner-Evanson, A., et al. "Honey promotes lower weight gain, adiposity, and triglycerides than sucrose in rats." *Nutrition Research* 31, no. 1 (January 2011): 55–60.

17. Worlds Healthiest Foods; www.whfoods.com

18. Katz, D. L., Doughty, K., Ali, A. "Cocoa and chocolate in human health and disease." *Antioxidants and redox signaling* 15, no. 10 (November 15, 2011): 2779–811. Epub 2011 Jun.

19. Si, H., Fu, Z., Babu, P. V., Zhen, W., Leroith, T., Meaney, M. P., Voelker, K. A., Jia, Z., Grange, R. W., Liu, D. "Dietary epicatechin promotes survival of obese diabetic mice and Drosophila melanogaster." *Journal of Nutrition* 141, no. 6 (June 2011): 1095–100. Epub 2011 Apr 27.

20. Morris, C. J., Fullick, S., Gregson, W., Clarke, N., Doran, D., MacLaren, D., Atkinson, G. "Paradoxical post-exercise responses of acylated ghrelin and leptin during a simulated night shift." *Chronobiology International* 27, no. 3 (May 2010): 590–605; and Broom, D. R., Stensel, D. J., Bishop, N. C., Burns, S. F., Miyashita, M. "Exercise-induced suppression of acylated ghrelin in humans." *Journal of Applied Physiology* 102, no. 6 (June 2007): 2165–71. Epub 2007 Mar 8.

21. Kirk, E. P., Donnelly, J. E., Smith, B. K., Honas, J., Lecheminant, J. D., Bailey, B. W., Jacobsen, D. J., Washburn, R. A. "Minimal resistance training improves daily energy expenditure and fat oxidation." *Medicine and Science in Sports and Exercise* 41, no. 5 (May 2009): 1122–9.

22. Whyte, L. J., Gill, J. M., Cathcart, A. J. "Effect of 2 weeks of sprint interval training on health-related outcomes in sedentary overweight/obese men." *Metabolism* 59, no. 10 (October 2010): 1421–8. Epub 2010 Feb 12.

Chapter 8

1. Wing, R. R., Phelan, S. "Long-term weight loss maintenance." *American Journal of Clinical Nutrition* 82, supplement no. 1 (July 2005): 222S–225S.

2. Ogden, J. "The correlates of long-term weight loss: a group comparison study of obesity." *International Journal of Obesity and Related Metabolic Disorders* 24, no. 8 (August 2000): 1018–25.

3. See note 2 above.

4. Dalle Grave, R., Calugi, S., Centis, E., El Ghoch, M., Marchesini, G. "Cognitive-behavioral strategies to increase the adherence to exercise in the management of obesity." *Journal of Obesity,* October 2011. Epub 2010 Oct 28.

5. Jakicic, J. M., Wing, R. R., Butler, B. A., Robertson, R. J. "Prescribing exercise in multiple short bouts versus one continuous bout: effects on adherence, cardiorespiratory fitness, and weight loss in overweight women." *International Journal of Obesity and Related Metabolic Disorders* 19, no. 12 (December 1995): 893–901.

6. Laddu, D., Dow, C., Hingle, M., Thomson, C., Going, S. "A review of evidence-based strategies to treat obesity in adults." *Nutrition in Clinical Practice* 26, no. 5 (October 2011): 512–25.

Index

Conversion Charts

ABBREVIATIONS

C	Celsius
cm	centimeter
F	Fahrenheit
fl oz	fluid ounce
ft	foot
g	gram
gal	gallon
in.	inch
kg	kilogram
L	liter
lb	pound
m	meter
mL	milliliter
mm	millimeter
oz	ounce
qt	quart
tbsp	tablespoon
tsp	teaspoon

TEASPOONS

⅛ tsp	0.5 mL
¼ tsp	1 mL
½ tsp	2 mL
¾ tsp	4 mL
1 tsp	5 mL
1½ tsp	7 mL
2 tsp	10 mL

TABLESPOONS

1 tbsp	15 mL
1½ tbsp	20 mL
2 tbsp	30 mL
3 tbsp	45 mL
4 tbsp	60 mL
5 tbsp	75 mL
6 tbsp	90 mL
8 tbsp	125 mL

WEIGHTS

1 oz	30 g
2 oz	60 g
3 oz	90 g
4 oz	125 g
5 oz	150 g
6 oz	175 g
8 oz	250 g
10 oz	300 g
12 oz	375 g
16 oz	500 g
32 oz	1 kg
¼ lb	125 g
½ lb	250 g
⅔ lb	300 g
¾ lb	375 g
1 lb	500 g
2 lb	1 kg
3 lb	1.5 kg

LENGTHS

¼ in.	5 mm
½ in.	1 cm
1 in.	2.5 cm
2 in.	5 cm
6 in.	15 cm
1 ft	30 cm

VOLUME

1 fl oz	30 mL
2 fl oz	50 mL
5 fl oz	150 mL
10 fl oz	300 mL
1 pint	500 mL
1 qt	1 L
1 gal	4 L
¼ cup	60 mL
⅓ cup	75 mL
½ cup	125 mL
⅔ cup	150 mL
¾ cup	175 mL
1 cup	250 mL
1¼ cups	300 mL
1½ cups	375 mL
2 cups	500 mL
4 cups	1 L
6 cups	1.5 L

OVEN TEMPERATURES

°F	°C
175°F	80°C
200°F	95°C
225°F	110°C
250°F	120°C
275°F	140°C
300°F	150°C
325°F	160°C
350°F	180°C
375°F	190°C
400°F	200°C
425°F	220°C
450°F	230°C
475°F	240°C
500°F	260°C

BAKING PANS

8 x 8 in.	20 x 20 cm
9 x 9 in.	22 x 22 cm
9 x 13 in.	22 x 33 cm
10 x 15 in.	25 x 38 cm
11 x 17 in.	28 x 43 cm
8 x 2 in. (round)	20 x 5 cm
9 x 2 in. (round)	22 x 5 cm
10 x 4½ in. (tube)	25 x 11 cm
8 x 4 x 3 in. (loaf)	20 x 10 x 7.5 cm
9 x 5 x 3 in. (loaf)	22 x 12.5 x 7.5 cm

CASSEROLE DISHES

Recipe calls for	Substitute
1 qt (4 cups)	900 mL
1½ qt (6 cups)	1.35 L
2–2½ qt (8–10 cups)	2.25 L
3 qt (12 cups)	2.7 L
4–5 qt (16–20 cups)	4.5 L

Want More Fat Releasing Food?

Look for *The Digest Diet Cookbook*, coming soon, which will feature 150 all-new recipes featuring the 13 fat releasing foods, including:

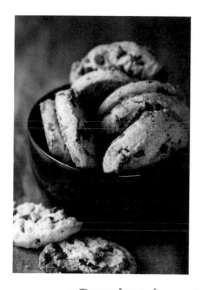

- **Grab-and-go breakfasts** such as Butternut Breakfast Bread and Mexican Breakfast Wraps
- **Comforting soups** such as Mom's Chicken Noodle Soup and Creamy Double-Mushroom Barley Soup
- **Hearty entrees** such as Eggplant Meatballs with Pasta, Pan-Seared Sirloin with Red Wine Sauce, and Crunchy Oven-Fried Chicken with Cajun Sweet Potato Fries
- **Versatile side dishes** and salads such as Old-School Spinach Salad, Honey Mustard Cabbage Slaw, and Barley Risotto with Collards
- **Decadent desserts** such as Strawberry Cheesecake Mouse and Chocolate Chocolate Chip Cookie

In addition, the cookbook will offer:

- **Guidelines** on how to mix and match recipes to create your own Digest Diet menus
- **Quick and easy tips** on organizing your kitchen to encourage fat releasing
- **Daily menus** for people who are vegetarian, dairy-free, or have other special needs

The Digest Diet Cookbook is all you need to lose weight and keep it off without sacrificing taste or convenience. Preorder it today!

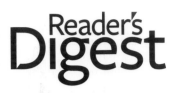
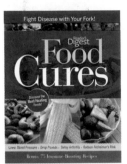
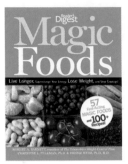
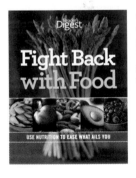
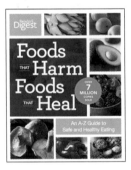
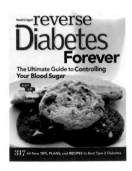
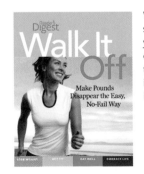